—— GET BACK ——
# YOUR SMILE,
—— TAKE BACK ——
# YOUR LIFE!

— GET BACK —

# YOUR SMILE,

— TAKE BACK —

# YOUR LIFE!

*how to artistically create*

## REMARKABLE

*dental results for the*

## REMARKABLE YOU

## DR. R. CRAIG MILLER

*Advantage.*

Published by Advantage, Charleston, South Carolina.
Member of Advantage Media Group.

ADVANTAGE is a registered trademark, and the Advantage colophon is a trademark of Advantage Media Group, Inc.

Printed in the United States of America.

10 9 8 7 6 5 4 3 2 1

ISBN: 978-1-64225-002-2
LCCN: 2019938207

Cover design by Megan Elger.
Layout design by Carly Blake.

This publication is designed to provide accurate and authoritative information in regard to the subject matter covered. It is sold with the understanding that the publisher is not engaged in rendering legal, accounting, or other professional services. If legal advice or other expert assistance is required, the services of a competent professional person should be sought.

Advantage Media Group is proud to be a part of the Tree Neutral® program. Tree Neutral offsets the number of trees consumed in the production and printing of this book by taking proactive steps such as planting trees in direct proportion to the number of trees used to print books. To learn more about Tree Neutral, please visit www.treeneutral.com.

Advantage Media Group is a publisher of business, self-improvement, and professional development books and online learning. We help entrepreneurs, business leaders, and professionals share their Stories, Passion, and Knowledge to help others Learn & Grow. Do you have a manuscript or book idea that you would like us to consider for publishing? Please visit advantagefamily.com or call 1.866.775.1696.

*To my patients that have trusted me with their dental health. To my parents for the DNA they have passed on to me which contains passion, drive, and humility. To Brenda—my loving wife— and our children. You complete me.*

# TABLE OF CONTENTS

FOREWORD . . . . . . . . . . . . . . . . . . . . . ix

INTRODUCTION . . . . . . . . . . . . . . . . . . 1

CHAPTER ONE . . . . . . . . . . . . . . . . . . 7
A GREAT SMILE IS YOUR GREATEST ASSET

CHAPTER TWO . . . . . . . . . . . . . . . . . . 19
THE COMPONENTS OF A GREAT SMILE

CHAPTER THREE . . . . . . . . . . . . . . . . . 29
NOSES ARE FOR BREATHING, MOUTHS ARE FOR EATING

CHAPTER FOUR . . . . . . . . . . . . . . . . . 45
THE FOUNDATION FOR A BEAUTIFUL SMILE

CHAPTER FIVE . . . . . . . . . . . . . . . . . . 61
ACHIEVING ESTHETIC EXCELLENCE
THROUGH DENTAL RESTORATION

CHAPTER SIX . . . . . . . . . . . . . . . . . . . 79
GETTING YOUR ORAL FUNCTION BACK

CHAPTER SEVEN. . . . . . . . . . . . . . . . . . . . 91

## ACHIEVING THE ULTIMATE OUTCOME

CHAPTER EIGHT. . . . . . . . . . . . . . . . . . 107

## WHAT MOTIVATES YOU?

CONCLUSION  . . . . . . . . . . . . . . . . . . . 115

ACKNOWLEDGMENTS . . . . . . . . . . . . . . 119

ABOUT THE AUTHOR . . . . . . . . . . . . . . 121

CONTACT US  . . . . . . . . . . . . . . . . . . 123

# FOREWORD

E very year I have the honor of interviewing applicants to the dental residency program at Newark Beth Israel Medical Center. To cut the tension, we may ask the prospective general practice resident in dentistry, "Why did you decide to become a dentist?" Every applicant can expect this question. The answer is almost always the same. "I wanted to enter a profession that marries my love for science, art, and people."

The young dentist we are interviewing is hoping that, over the course of their career, they will be able to successfully marry these three passions. Having a love for something does not necessarily mean that you have the talent, attitude, and work ethic to be successful as a dentist or any other professional.

In the end, how can we measure anyone's "success" as a dentist? What metrics should we use? How do we know that, over time, any dentist has been truly able to marry his or her passion for science, art, and working with people? The answer for me is they are a "difference maker." I believe Dr. R. Craig Miller is a difference maker. I have witnessed how he makes a difference in the lives he touches.

Dr. Miller's knowledge of the science of dentistry is on display when he lectures and informally teaches our residents. It is evident whenever we "talk dentistry" or attend continuing education courses together.

He is a true artist. The esthetic results of his cases are marvels. When I look at his cases, sometimes all I can say is "Wow."

Communication (people) skills are another area where Craig excels. In a successful dental practice, it is the dentist's love of their patients that can sometimes be the most important element to the success of the practice. The feeling should and will be mutual. As much as Dr. Miller loves his patients, his patients love Dr. Miller.

Is Dr. Miller a difference maker? The answer is a resounding *yes*. While it is obvious to his friends and colleagues, it is most profound in his patients. Dr. Miller uses his experience and perspective to make a difference in the lives of the people that he serves and sets an example for those who are looking to him for leadership and guidance. Changing a patient's life by eliminating long-term pain or changing a patient's smile is life changing. He has made a difference in many of his patients. Dr. Miller has married his love of science, art, and people. He deserves the title of "difference maker," and in reading this book you too will find out why this is true.

**Russ Bergman, DMD**
Vice Chair and General Practice Residency Program Director
Department of Dentistry
Newark Beth Israel Medical Center

# INTRODUCTION

*"The happiness of life is made up of little things—a smile, a helping hand, a caring heart, a word of praise, a moment of shared laughter. We are most alive in those moments. Savor them all!"*

**—Dan Zadra**

As I approached my thirtieth year of changing lives one smile at a time, I found myself reflecting on the goals that I had set and achieved.

That's what it really takes to regain dental harmony: setting and achieving goals. That includes watching what you eat and getting regular exercise. While I live and breathe that belief today, that's a much different mind-set from the one I had when I was younger. All through college, I didn't care what I ate. It didn't matter then because I jogged four miles every other day and the weight stayed off. But after a while, I became bored with jogging—life got busier, and before long, being overweight became the norm.

What I learned from that experience was the value of moderation. I began watching what I ate and doing different kinds of exercise on different days. That led to biking, my favorite low-impact aerobic activity. I got the biking bug after riding with a friend, Steve. Before long, I was biking twenty-five miles a day on average. I loved being outside on a beautiful day, biking over rolling hills, and passing waterfalls and rippling brooks, horse stables, vegetable farms, and beautiful homes.

I set goals with each ride to try to improve my performance; some goals were easier to reach than others. Finally, in 2002, I decided to ride from New York City to Washington, DC, in honor of the lives lost in the World Trade Center attack a year earlier. I would need to ride around one hundred miles per day for three straight days, and I had three months to train.

Now, I'm no world-class biker. I am a full-time dentist with a chronic lower back condition. I also have asthma, which makes endurance and maintaining breathing strength over long periods of time a challenge. To succeed in this biking marathon, I needed to be in exceptional shape, not just good shape, and I needed to overcompensate for my shortcomings.

I developed a training regimen that included going to the gym at five o'clock, four mornings a week to lift light weights and do various low-impact aerobics. That sometimes included spin classes, which are instructor-led, stationary-cycling sessions with music. In the weeks before the big ride, I would do some "hill work" in the evening: I would ride up and down hills as fast as I could, over and over, before heading for home.

Eating right was especially important in getting ready for the ride. Junk food and sodas were out. Fruits, vegetables, and egg whites were in. Today, even when I'm not preparing for any kind of endurance challenge, I still try to stay fit and eat a healthy diet, since both lead to healthy living.

As one of my mentors, Tony Robbins, writes in his book *Awaken the Giant Within: How to Take Immediate Control of your Mental, Emotional, Physical and Financial Destiny*, "The failure of most individuals to grasp the difference between fitness and health is what causes them to experience the frustration of working out religiously and still having the same five to ten pounds stubbornly clinging to their midsection." Being disciplined and understanding the value of goal-setting and the difference between fitness and health helped me prepare for what was, for me, a world-class biking challenge.

September came and 1,500 riders donned red, white, and blue shirts and gathered at a street adjacent to Ground Zero. Greg LeMond, a three-time Tour de France champion, was there to spur us on. That three-hundred-mile challenge would be my Tour.

On day one, the terrain was mostly flat. On day two, I rode for one hundred miles before the ride became more challenging, especially since I ran out of water. My friend Steve was also having a tough go of it, so we motivated each other to keep going. When we reached the finish line on day three, I felt I had just conquered the world. I overcame my body's shortcomings to do something incredible that helped my body, mind, and soul. Words cannot describe all of the complex emotions I experienced at the end of the journey, but meeting that challenge made me feel I could accomplish almost anything I put my mind to.

For some people, getting back their smiles elicits the same response. After the journey of time, effort, and money that it can take to regain dental harmony, a beautiful smile in the mirror can be the reward for achieving something truly wonderful. Keeping that smile then becomes the goal, but one that is well worth the effort because it can make you feel great, eat better, and keep your body sound.

## MORE THAN DRILL AND FILL

From the start, I have always been interested in being more than a drill-and-fill dentist. To ensure that, I've always pursued continuing education beyond dental school at the University of Medicine and Dentistry of New Jersey, and I did an advanced general dental practice residency at Mount Sinai Hospital in Manhattan. In fact, early on, I dove into the cosmetic and implant disciplines of dentistry because I liked the art of cosmetic dentistry and the surgical side of implantology. In addition to my general and advanced dentistry schooling, I completed three years of intensive, hands-on oral implantology training and trained in treating the entire system of facial joints, muscles, and teeth.

In my practice, I never wanted to be beholden to insurance companies that dictate what kind of dentistry patients can receive. When I first began practicing, good esthetics and implantology weren't covered by most insurance companies. So, from the start, I have always had a fee-for-service practice. That has allowed me to approach patients' mouths as, essentially, blank canvasses. By not being bound to insurance company rules for payment and treatment, the patients and I have more control over how we can turn their mouths into healthy, fully functioning, beautiful works of art.

You see, no matter how much education dentists have, no matter what kind of artistry they produce, no matter how well they treat their patients, dental insurers pay every practitioner the same amount for any particular service—across the board. Even if I were to create a better crown, or make a mouth more stable, or create a better smile, I would get the same amount of compensation as any other practitioner. But dentistry is not an even playing field, no matter what insurance companies would have you believe. It's similar to choosing a restaurant: there are five-star restaurants, chain restaurants such as

Chili's and Red Robin, and fast food restaurants such as McDonald's and Wendy's. As a consumer, you definitely get to choose the quality of what you pay for. When you are serious about your health, you need the most qualified and experienced professionals on your team.

Since I don't want to play insurance games, I bring a different dental experience to the table, one that places education, customer service, and artistry at the forefront. Once my patients understand that, they can't wait to get started on treatment. It's a philosophy that has worked well for my patients for thirty years and counting and continues to enable me to provide remarkable dentistry at the highest level.

In fact, over time, my view has helped grow my practice into what I call a hybrid dental practice, where complementing services include general, cosmetic, restorative, and surgical dentistry along with solutions for sleep apnea and temporomandibular joint (TMJ) disorder.

I offer these services today, in part because I used to refer work to doctors who specialized in certain dental disciplines. But when patients came back to me, they were not always happy. Sometimes that was because of the service they had received. Sometimes it was because of the work that had been done. The dental office is not usually anyone's favorite place to go, but it's a win for my patients when they don't have to go elsewhere for some of their dental needs. While I offer several services under one roof, I never wanted to become a jack of all trades and master of none. So, I don't aim to be all things to all patients, but I endeavor to be the best in those additional services that I do provide.

## MASTERY IN YOUR LIFE

I titled this book *Get Back Your Smile, Take Back Your Life*. However, what does it really mean to "get back your smile"? In the literal sense, it's turning stained, broken, and yellow teeth, into white, straightened, and beautiful teeth. In the figurative sense, it's about what happens once the beautiful smile is obtained.

How else do you take back your life? By taking action and executing mastery in your life: at home, in business, with your family, and with your health. Being healthy and smiling at the world can change everything. Once you take control of your smile and your health, you can master other areas of your life.

Another mentor of mine, Kevin Kowalke, introduced me to the book *Mastery: The Keys to Success and Long-Term Fulfillment*, in which George Leonard writes, "What is mastery? … It brings rich rewards, yet is not really a goal or a destination, but rather a process, a journey … Mastery isn't reserved for the super talented, or even for those who are fortunate enough to have gotten an early start. It's available to anyone who is willing to get on the path and stay on it."

What I hope you find in this book is that a great smile, a healthy mouth, and a good night's sleep can be the first step on your path to mastering your life. In the pages ahead, I will discuss, among other topics, the power of a great smile, the range of effective treatments that exist today for creating a great smile, and the role of breathing well in getting a good night's sleep, which is key to overall health.

I wrote this book for adults who desire to take care of themselves, to find ways to make themselves feel better mentally and physically. Getting back your smile is certainly a challenge for many people. But taking the dental plunge can be the first step to regaining your smile—and your overall health. Yes, life is a series of challenges that can lead to great rewards. I hope that the information I'm sharing in the pages ahead will inspire you to set goals to improve and empower yourself to take back your health and to always smile.

# CHAPTER ONE

# A GREAT SMILE IS YOUR GREATEST ASSET

person's smile is a very powerful asset in our culture today. A patient of mine, Karin, knew the power of a great smile, which is why she came into my office to have me evaluate her teeth to see what could be improved.

In her midthirties, Karin decided it was time to finally do something about her gummy smile, which is when more than the normal amount of gum shows during a smile, making the teeth appear shorter and adding years to a person. In addition to showing too much gum, her gum line was also uneven, making her teeth appear crooked and irregularly shaped.

Although she was a happy person, she had begun to feel self-conscious about the condition of her less-than-ideal smile, so she would often cover her mouth with her hand when she laughed. She came to me, hoping to improve some of what she saw in the mirror, and she felt certain that a better smile would help her feel more confident in how she greeted the world.

Interestingly, Karin worked in a pharmacy that was adjacent to a cosmetic dental office, but she chose to see me because other patients had told her about their successes, and she had visited my website and seen the before-and-after results. That convinced her that we were the best fit for her needs and wants.

After a thorough examination of her mouth, teeth, and gums, along with x-ray imaging to look at the underlying structures of her mouth, I was happy to share with Karin that we could perform corrective procedures that would give her the smile she desired and deserved.

## A GREAT SMILE SPEAKS VOLUMES

A great smile says a lot about you. My friend and mentor Scott Manning, MBA, says, "The power of communication is a great smile." Think about that. Your smile is the first thing people see when they meet you, and the main feature they remember after meeting you.[1] A nice, healthy smile literally attracts people to you the way a work of art attracts people in a museum or art gallery. When people are attracted to you and your smile, they will take you more seriously and listen more closely. In fact, in a study involving peoples' reactions to a series of photos of people, researchers found the following data.

- Nearly half (45 percent) viewed a person with straight teeth as more likely to find employment than an applicant with crooked teeth.

- More than half (58 percent) believed a person with straight teeth was more successful and wealthier.

---

1   "First Impressions Are Everything: New Study Confirms People with Straight Teeth Are Perceived as More Successful, Smarter and Having More Dates," Invisalign, April 19, 2012, accessed March 7, 2018, https://www.prnewswire.com/news-releases/first-impressions-are-everything-new-study-confirms-people-with-straight-teeth-are-perceived-as-more-successful-smarter-and-having-more-dates-148073735.html.

- Nearly three quarters (73 percent) felt a person with a nice smile was more trust worthy than a well-dressed person.

A national survey also found that people looking for a partner rated teeth as the top must-have, noting it as an indicator of overall hygiene.[2]

Let's face it. A smile is empowering. It says, "Here I am, world. Take notice." And when others notice, they see and hear you more clearly. When you smile, the world smiles back at you.

A great smile lowers people's anxiety about their appearance. It heightens self-esteem. It creates a feeling of self-confidence.

A smile affects how you behave: how you sit, stand, greet people, and converse with them. The lack of a smile puts you in a state of mind that is disempowering and can even lower your level of performance.

## WHAT MAKES A SMILE GREAT?

A great smile is more than just beautiful, white teeth. A great smile is also about the shape of the teeth and how they come together in what's known as the bite. It is about the relation of the teeth and gums to the lips. And it features healthy gums that are pink and firm, not red and inflamed or swollen and bleeding.

In short, a great smile is one in which all of its components are in harmony, and one that leaves a positive and lasting impression.

A smile in the morning, upon waking, is a good indicator of what's going on behind the teeth. Happy, healthy people smile because their mouth looks good and functions well. A really great smile is also lifesaving: it functionally enhances better oral and overall health by allowing the wearer to eat and breathe better.

---

2    Sharon Jayson, "What Singles Want: Survey Looks at Attraction, Turnoffs," *USA Today*, February 5, 2013, accessed June 20, 2018, https://www.usatoday.com/story/news/nation/2013/02/04/singles-dating-attraction-facebook/1878265.

Take, for instance, a mouth that has an upper jaw developed too far forward, into what's known as an overbite, where the upper front teeth envelop the lower front teeth. That can limit the development of the lower jaw and create an environment in which the teeth are crowded and there is not enough room for the tongue. As a result, the tongue will function in ways that wreak havoc on the position of the teeth, make it more difficult to swallow, and can force the tongue into the back of the throat, which can close off the airway. That's a problem when it happens during sleep and, over time, can even affect the shape of the smile and the face. When people can't breathe through their noses, the position their mouth takes to accommodate that closed breathing passage can, ultimately, cause the face to elongate. Correcting the breathing issue in a younger, still-developing patient can help the face begin to shorten up and round out a bit, making it look and breathe a little healthier.

These are just some of the conditions that make for a less-than-ideal mouth. I will discuss them further in the chapters ahead.

## THE LINK TO OVERALL HEALTH

People who have unhealthy teeth often have poor overall health. Granted, that may be simply because they don't take care of themselves or their teeth. But it may also be because their teeth prevent them from eating as well as they could. Conversely, it may be that they don't eat healthy food, which has contributed to poor oral health.

Whatever the reason, there are definite correlations between oral disease and the overall health of the body. Some of the leading causes of death identified by the Centers for Disease Control and Prevention (CDC) can be connected to problems with the mouth. They include heart disease, cancer, chronic lower respiratory diseases, stroke, and

Alzheimer's disease.[3] Poor oral health can also complicate diabetes and can raise the risk of preterm birth in pregnant women.[4]

Periodontal disease can cause people to have a

- 24 to 35 percent higher chance of developing plaque in their coronary arteries;

- 4.5 percent greater chance of experiencing a stroke;

- 2.6 percent higher risk of developing Alzheimer's disease;

- 93 percent likelihood of developing diabetes;

- 62 percent higher chance of pancreatic cancer;

- greater risk for problems such as bronchitis, asthma, and emphysema; and

- 30 to 50 percent higher risk of having a preterm or low-birth-weight baby.[5]

So, it's not just teeth and gums; your whole body can be at risk if you let your dental health go. The problems in the mouth can lead to inflammation and infections that can affect the entire body.

## DENTAL CARE IS KEY

As the body ages, it is less able to deal with disease and recover from the negative effects of oxidative stress.[6] Oxidative stress is the damaging effect of free radicals, which are harmful molecules in the body's cells,

---

3    "Deaths and Mortality," CDC, accessed June 21, 2018, https://www.cdc.gov/nchs/fastats/deaths.htm.

4    Jamie Toop, "The Practice of Oral-Systemic Health," *AGD Impact* 46, no. 2 (February 2018): 12–16, https://www.agd.org/2/publications/impact/issues/2018/feb/html5.

5    Ibid.

6    Uche Ochiatu, "Adding More Life to Your Years," *The Profitable Dentist*, accessed June 20, 2018, http://tpdmag.com/fall-2017.

---

resulting from breathing in and using oxygen.

Bad bacteria are the primary drivers of the problems in the mouth. Without proper oral care—a good regimen of brushing, flossing, eating healthier foods, and having good levels of vitamins and minerals in the body—good bacteria in the mouth can turn to harmful bacteria, which can lead to tooth decay. Enzymes in saliva that kill the decaying type of bacteria on the teeth can weaken against the "bugs" that attack gum tissue and bone. When bad bacteria infect the tissues surrounding teeth, they cause inflammation. If those bacteria remain on the teeth, plaque and, ultimately, tartar (or calculus) form. That can spread below the gum line, where only a dental professional can remove it.[7]

Oral hygiene has a direct impact on the mouth's microbiome, the balance of organisms that keep decay at bay. Without good oral hygiene, the mouth is at risk for developing periodontal disease. Periodontitis is the leading cause of tooth loss in adults.[8] In fact, the CDC estimates that nearly half of adults (47.2 percent) age thirty or older suffer from some form of periodontal disease, and incidences of it increase with age: nearly three-fourths (70.1 percent) of adults age sixty-five or older have it.[9]

Excess sugar is one of the primary culprits of plaque. Bad bacteria in the mouth feed off sugar. The more sugar in the diet, the higher the propensity for dental and periodontal breakdown. In chapter 4, I'll talk more about how diet and nutrition affect the teeth and mouth.

Regular and correct brushing and flossing are key to oral and

---

7    "Periodontal Disease," Centers for Disease Control and Prevention, accessed June 21, 2018, https://www.cdc.gov/oralhealth/periodontal_disease/index.htm.

8    "Periodontal (Gum) Disease," National Institute of Dental and Craniofacial Research, accessed June 21, 2018, https://www.nidcr.nih.gov/research/data-statistics/periodontal-disease.

9    "Periodontal Disease," Centers for Disease Control and Prevention, accessed June 21, 2018, https://www.cdc.gov/oralhealth/periodontal_disease/index.htm.

overall health. Patients who have good oral hygiene spend less on health care overall.[10] Proper brushing and flossing can turn back the clock on gum disease in many cases, helping to avoid further inflammation and, eventually, tooth loss.

## LIFE GETS BUSY

As humans, we get caught up in life's twists and turns. My patients often tell me that they put their kids first: the kids get the braces, the kids take the summer trips, the kids have all these sporting activities. Parents, especially, just get caught up in their daily family life. When it isn't family, it's work. Everything else takes a back seat to self-care. Then, after the kids graduate from high school and go off to college, the parents start to notice things happening in their mouth. They've spent their life thus far taking care of someone else, but now, they decide, it's their turn. It's time for them to do something for themselves.

Poor dental health can stem from any number of traps in life, a subject researched in-depth by Jeffery E. Young and Janet S. Klosko. "Lifetraps," as the researchers term them, are "negative behavior patterns" that can develop in childhood, depending on how a child is raised, and then carry over into adulthood. The researchers identified eleven traps that subconsciously influence how a person thinks, feels, and acts.[11]

1. **Abandonment**. When children are abandoned by someone very close to them, they develop feelings of distrust or of being unsafe.

---

10  Shawn F. Kane, "The Effects of Oral Health on Systemic Health," *General Dentistry* 6, no. 6 (November/December 2017): 30–34.

11  "11 Traps in Life," myempoweredworld.com, May 24, 2012, accessed June 20, 2018, http://myempoweredworld.com/personal-growth/lifetraps.

2. **Abuse.** Children who are abused by someone very close to them also develop feelings of distrust or being unsafe.

3. **Emotional deprivation.** People can experience a sense of disconnect on an emotional or intimate level.

4. **Social exclusion.** This is another type of disconnect that people can experience on a social or societal level.

5. **Dependency**. Children who don't learn to be self-sufficient and independent develop a sense of dependency.

6. **Vulnerability.** A child whose parent worries about disasters or being harmed may develop a sense of vulnerability.

7. **Defectiveness.** A child who is not shown appreciation or is excessively criticized may develop a sense of defectiveness.

8. **Failure.** Children may develop a sense of failure if they feel they lack talent or are not smart enough to succeed.

9. **Subjugation.** People who need to constantly accommodate others' wishes are subjugating themselves to the control of others.

10. **Perfection.** An unrelenting need to strive for perfection can lead a person to feel that life is empty or joyless.

11. **Entitlement.** People who have a sense of entitlement were spoiled as a child.

What's important is to recognize these traps and how they affect your life—and your oral health. They shape behavior by creating almost a circuit in the brain that makes it think that the treatment is acceptable. Let's take, for instance, self-esteem. If your parents made you feel inadequate as a youngster, you grow up always wanting to try to prove to everybody that you're adequate. You might also be wired to think that you're going to fail at everything you do. That includes taking care of your teeth. If people believe they are going to fail, they can undermine any attempt to do what's best for them. If they think they are not worthy of a great smile, then they won't go after it.

But there is a way to break that circuitry. One way is to just do it. If you want to lose weight, take control of your health. If you want a nicer smile, do your homework (brush and floss) and get professional help (in the form of dental care). When you do positive things for yourself, you can break the feeling of failure.

Getting your teeth treated is a very easy step in the right direction. Once you have great dental work done and you see those results, you can then begin to feel worthy of greater things. Once you have a great smile, you can take it out into the world, and who knows where you can go with it. Maybe you'll find ways to change the world for the better.

## GOOD ORAL HEALTH IS A TEAM SPORT

When it comes to having a great smile, dental treatment alone offers no guarantees for the long term—not without help from you, the patient. Successful outcomes rely on the patient to be a member of the care team.

We use our skill, expertise, and technology to create great smiles. We educate patients on what they need to do to get the outcome they desire. But it's their responsibility to get their desired outcome and then to keep their new smile in the best condition possible. What patients do when they're not in the dental office determines their long-term outcome. That includes proper home care and getting regular cleanings at their dentist's office.

Unfortunately, Dolly is an example of what can happen when home care and follow-up visits are ignored. She came to me for help with her smile because it was driving her low self-esteem, and that was keeping her in a job in which she felt trapped. Finally, she woke up one day and said to herself, "Enough. I'm going to get my teeth fixed, get a new job, and get a better life for myself and my family." And she did just that. But even before I placed her implants and veneers, I told her, "Dolly, it's up to you to keep your mouth in tip-top shape, because just like natural teeth, implants can also have problems." Whether patients have one or twenty implants, we strongly recommend they come in for what we call re-care appointments every three or four months, rather than once or twice a year, because implants are a little more susceptible to bacteria than natural tooth structure. It takes ideal home care, plus coming in to the dental office for those regular "maintenance" checkups to ensure that implanted teeth stay strong and in place.

At first, Dolly was so delighted with her smile that she took great care of it. She even followed through on her plans to get a new job and better life. Then, she stopped coming into the office for five years. She was very healthy when she stopped coming in, but five years later, she showed up with a dental implant in her hand. Since she was given specific instructions upfront, she knew that the failure of the implant was her own doing since she had failed to keep her mouth in tip-top shape.

Recently, I had esthetic work done on my own smile. It made me feel better knowing that I looked better. Also, I knew the importance of keeping my smile healthy because of the susceptibility of restorative dentistry to bacteria. Before my cosmetic makeover, I flossed once a day. Today, I floss two or three times daily to keep my smile looking great and to keep from having the treatment redone.

## A GREAT SMILE IS AN INVESTMENT

A great smile is more than investment in dental work; it's an investment in your future.

I continue to look for advances in dentistry that will lengthen the longevity of every patient's esthetic and functional investment. Recently, for instance, I have begun advocating the use of a water flosser in addition to brushing, flossing, and mouthwash. I have used one ever since I tried it out and found that it removed more debris, even after I thought I had done a great job of cleaning my mouth.

Your teeth are meant to be with you for life. That's the goal. But if you lose a tooth, we have solutions that can look and feel similar to your natural teeth. Whether it's an implant-supported tooth, or a natural tooth, it's our objective to help every all our patients keep their oral health at its best.

## KARIN'S OUTCOME: LESS GUM, MORE TEETH

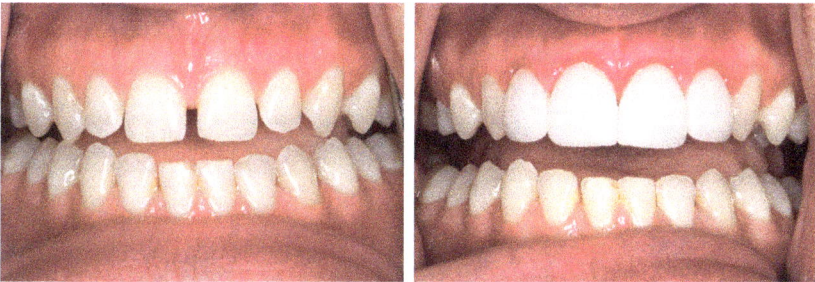

BEFORE          AFTER

Remember Karin at the beginning of the chapter? Well, after I performed a gum lift on her, also known as gum contouring, her smile exploded. A gum lift involves sculpting excess and uneven tissue around the teeth to make the gums symmetrical and proportionate to the teeth and overall smile. Gum contouring is a quick and relatively painless way to create a more symmetrical gum line to improve the overall appearance of a smile.

The procedure was done in a single visit under a local anesthetic and using a state-of-the-art laser, which provided precise results. The laser also lessens discomfort and decreases recovery time. Karin had a little discomfort with the procedure, for which she took over-the-counter medication. Her soreness and swelling subsided within a week, and she was left with a beaming, beautiful smile.

# Quick Quiz

1. What are three features of a great smile?

2. What are five diseases that can increase in risk with poor oral hygiene?

3. Name three traps in life that keep people in a negative state of mind.

4. Why is proper home care important to long-term success with cosmetic dentistry?

# CHAPTER TWO

# THE COMPONENTS OF A GREAT SMILE

M arissa was in her midtwenties when she came to me wanting "larger, straighter, and whiter" front teeth. She was so self-conscious about the condition of her teeth that she smiled with her mouth closed. She had broken her two upper front teeth when she was in second grade and had veneers to correct the problem. But over time, the treatment had not held up well and left her with an unattractive smile.

When I removed the old veneer, the amount of tooth left was not sufficient for another veneer, but it was ideal for a ceramic crown, or what many dentists refer to as a 360-degree laminate since it wraps around the tooth.

I took molds of her upper and lower jaws in a bite and then recreated her smile in wax on a dental model to make the teeth look esthetically pleasing. Known as a diagnostic wax-up, the model helped me figure out exactly how much gum tissue and bone to remove to get just the right amount of tooth exposure. It also let Marissa see what her finished smile would look like even before we began her treatment.

The wax-up becomes the blueprint for the final result.

Marissa also had an impacted wisdom tooth and several cavities in other teeth, which we corrected to bring her to optimal dental health.

Luckily, Marissa came in to have her dental issues addressed before they became compounded even more by the natural affects of aging.

Let's look at the progression of problems in the mouth through the years.

## A CHRONOLOGY OF DENTAL CARE

Health is a moving target, which is evident from dental health changes at different ages.

**The twenties**. At this age, young adults are often on their own for the first time in their lives, and they must take responsibility for their own oral care. That can take a little getting used to, resulting in a few cavities. But at this age, their younger bodies are still able to fend off disease, which includes gingivitis, or swelling and redness of the gums, an early sign of gum disease. Early gingivitis, including light bleeding of the gums, can often be reversed with better oral hygiene (regular brushing and flossing), and regular visits to the dentist.

**The thirties**. As young adults trying to make their way in the working world, people at this age may begin to feel the effects of stress on their teeth. Over time, activities such as clenching and grinding as well as daily chewing can create craze lines in teeth. Teeth that have had fillings for a while start to break down and weaken around the supporting tooth structure. Just as a pebble hitting a windshield does, a crack in a tooth can spread toward the nerve, requiring a crown to keep the crack from worsening. But young adults building a family in this decade may also find themselves putting off their own care for the sake of their child's care, delaying much-needed treatment of decay and other problems.

**The forties**. This is when we begin to see problems resulting from care not being taken earlier. Patients who are forty-something ask all the time, "Why is this happening now?" Usually, it is just the accumulation of not taking enough care at other critical junctures. If our bodies at twenty-something were to revolt, we would see the results of poor health sooner. While younger bodies are more tolerant of imbalances in the mouth, by the time people reach their forties, undermined tooth structure can lead to cracks, onlays, and crowns.

**The fifties**. Tooth loss can begin because of periodontal disease, which occurs when gingivitis isn't treated. In periodontal disease, the gums separate from the teeth and form spaces where bacteria, infection, and inflammation can set in. Left untreated, the bone and tissues holding the tooth in place will, eventually, break down. In time, the patient may lose the tooth.

Older teeth show more wear and tear as well. I'm writing this book in my midfifties. I just broke a tooth, the second one I've broken since I turned fifty. Both teeth were upper left premolars that had no fillings, no decay, and no previous dental treatment other than cleanings. It was simply a matter of wear and tear. As a person gets older, teeth just give up under all the chewing and clenching. Both teeth were fractured so badly that I had to have them extracted and bone grafted. Welcome to the fifties and the miracle of dental implants.

With age, the body becomes much less tolerant of the imbalances. It's important to take care of younger teeth to help avoid problems in older age. However, even if people let their teeth go, treatments and procedures today can help give them a healthier foundation that can then be built on.

# THE ANATOMY OF THE MOUTH

Teeth are, of course, the tools we use to chew food, but there is more to teeth than just the hard, white structure that we see. Let me share with you some basic anatomy of the mouth.

**Enamel** is the hard, protective exterior of the tooth. It is a protective shell that is exposed inside your mouth, or the translucent white part of the tooth that people see when they look at your smile.

**The clinical crown of a tooth** is composed of enamel and is the part of the tooth not covered by the gums. The crown of each tooth determines its function. Molars in the back of the mouth have a larger, flatter surface to use in grinding. Incisors in the front of the mouth have sharp edges to use in cutting.

**Dentin** is an inner layer of the tooth just below the enamel. Dentin separates the enamel from the pulp of the tooth. Dentin, while still considered a hard surface, is softer than enamel and very susceptible to decay.

**Pulp** is the softer interior of the tooth. The pulp of the tooth houses the nerves of the tooth and the blood vessels that supply nutrients.

**Roots**. Each tooth has roots, which are the part of the tooth that lives below the gum line.

**Cementum** is the hard surface of the tooth that covers the roots below the gum line. Cementum is similar in hardness to dentin and, as you might expect by its name, it cements the tooth to the jawbone.

**Gums** are the soft, pink tissues that conceal the roots of each tooth.

**Sulcus** is the space between the teeth and gums that is roughly two to three millimeters in depth. When the gums are not healthy, plaque can enter the sulcus and cause it to expand and inflame the gums, creating what's known as a periodontal pocket. Plaque in this area of the mouth can even eat away at the underlying bone.

When all of these components in the mouth are in harmony, there is good oral health. Let's look at some problems in the mouth that cause disharmony.

## HARMONY IN THE MOUTH

Healthy gums and bone are essential for beautiful teeth. When parts of the mouth start breaking down, not only do esthetics suffer, but the damage can lead to pain and, ultimately, to greater expense. The goal of treatment is to restore symmetry, balance, and health. What does that mean?

One idea of the perfect smile is based on a concept known as the golden proportion, which is, essentially, a definition of beauty based on mathematical calculations and items found in nature. Flowers, plants, seashells, and animals exhibit the mathematically ideal, golden proportion.

In humans, the golden proportion refers to an ideal ratio of facial measurements to define beauty. Those measurements take into account, for instance, the distance from the center of the pupil to the bottom of the teeth to the bottom of the chin. The golden proportion can also be applied to the mouth in proportion to the rest of the face, the length from the outer edges to the upper ridges of the lips, and the width of the center tooth to the width of the second tooth.[12] According to this concept, when the mouth and the body are in golden proportion, they are healthier and functioning normally.

---

12    Gary Meisner, "The Human Face and the Golden Ratio," The Golden Number, May 31, 2012, https://www.goldennumber.net/face.

Some dentists propose the use of the golden proportion as a way of helping to determine the ideal size and shape of teeth and their relation to the other teeth in the mouth.[13] When combined with other considerations such as tooth length, position, and plane or angle, the golden proportion can act as a guideline for preparing and fabricating restorative teeth.[14]

While there are ideal proportions, what's most important is to consider each patient's individual ideal. Every patient's face has a different shape and different contours, so the last thing I want is every patient walking around with the same smile. That's why treatments are not cookie-cutter. Every patient's treatment is tailored to that individual's specific needs, wants, and golden proportion.

## Problems of Disharmony

**Teeth**. In an esthetic smile, small variations in symmetry are acceptable. However, the two upper front teeth, known as the maxillary central incisors, must have complete bilateral symmetry since they are the dominant teeth in the smile. If one central incisor is wider or longer than the other, the eyes view that as asymmetry. The eyes are confused because they do not know which of the two upper front teeth to focus on.

Other elements necessary to creating a great smile include creating unique contours to the teeth and the patient's smile. These individualzed contours must fit the patient's personality, accentuate the curve of the lip, and blend with the unique facial features.

Beyond esthetics, health issues such as tooth decay, known in the dental profession as dental caries, can create disharmony in the mouth.

---

13   Dino Javaheri and Sara Shahnavaz, "Utilizing the Concept of the Golden Proportion," *Dentistry Today* 21, no. 6 (June 21, 2002), http://www.dentistrytoday.com/restorative-134/1889--sp-1971672447.

14   Ibid.

When bacteria fester on the surface nooks and crannies of the teeth, or the pits and fissures on and between the teeth, they create acids that eat away the enamel. When the toxins reach the dentin, you may feel sensitivity to cold and sometimes to heat, but you do not have to have thermal sensitivity to have decay. Sometimes decay can even act as an insulator to prevent sensitivity to cold. Once decay penetrates into the pulp, where the nerves live, then sensitivity to cold and heat lets you know that the nerve is infected and traumatized by decay. Catching the problem early enough may allow the problem to be reversed, but if the nerve becomes infected, it must be removed via root canal therapy.

**Occlusion or bite**. In the ideal mouth, the upper and lower teeth come together at the same time during a bite. If the bite is off, then harmony is disturbed. A misaligned bite, also known as malocclusion, could lead to loosening or breakage of the teeth, gum recession, and/ or TMJ problems and pain.

**Gingiva (gums)**. Gums must also have symmetry for there to be harmony in the mouth. If the gum height is lower on one upper middle tooth and higher on the adjacent tooth, as was the case with the asymmetrical teeth I mentioned earlier, the eyes get confused as to which gum height to focus on, creating an uncomfortable response in the mind.

There are two types of gum tissue in the mouth. One type is attached to teeth and bone and surrounds the necks of the teeth. The other is loose and movable and not attached to teeth and bone. You can usually find this type of tissue as the gums get closer to the cheeks. Ideally, there should be three millimeters of attached gum tissue, and all gum tissue should be a healthy pink. The eyes aren't accustomed to seeing red gums. That's a flag signaling disharmony in the mouth.

Gum tissue needs saliva to stay healthy. As mentioned in chapter

1, saliva helps remove plaque and keeps it from building up. Without saliva, plaque begins to accumulate on teeth and causes the gums to become irritated, red, and swollen, signs of inflammation or infection.

Even healthy gum tissue naturally recedes with age. That can expose the cementum (root surface of the tooth) and cause sensitivity to cold.

**Parafunction.** A habitual mouth movement that can't be controlled is parafunctional. Behaviors commonly considered parafunctional include bruxism (clenching or grinding), excessive gum chewing, and lip or fingernail biting. Parafunction is, of course, detrimental to a great smile. We dentists cannot alleviate parafunctional habits. For example, if patients grind their teeth, we cannot stop the parafunctional grinding, but we can slow down the aggressive wear on the teeth caused by the grinding by creating an appliance for the patient to wear during sleep, which is when most grinding occurs. Patients can then bite down and grind on the appliance instead of on their teeth.

**Breathing issues.** Problems with breathing can also lead to smile disharmony. If you're not breathing through your nose, you're breathing through your mouth. If you're breathing through your mouth, you're going to get dry mouth. In the absence of saliva, as I mentioned earlier, decay can begin to take hold of the teeth. Scalloped edges on the tongue are another sign that a patient may have breathing issues. Scalloping occurs when the jaw is too narrow to house the tongue. The next chapter is devoted to looking at the connection between oral health and sleep. First, however, let's look at some of the results we've had thus far with Marissa's treatment for oral esthetics and function.

## MARISSA'S SMILE

To restore Marissa's gummy smile and replace her prior dental treatment, I performed a crown-lengthening procedure to expose more of the natural tooth. That procedure involved trimming up the gum tissue to raise it higher on the teeth and contouring it to be attractive. The procedure requires a local anesthetic, but afterward, any discomfort is usually relieved with over-the-counter pain relievers.

Marissa's restoration also involved the extraction of a wisdom tooth, filling cavities with tooth-colored composite resin, and whitening teeth. Yet, one of the real challenges in her case was matching three veneers with one crown on the front teeth. Her upper four front teeth were shaped to receive porcelain veneers on three teeth along with a porcelain crown on the front tooth that was badly broken from a fall when she was only two years old. After we placed her temporary veneers and crown, I handed her a mirror. When she saw her new smile, she began to cry happy tears.

Upon completing the esthetics of her mouth, we will review her sleep situation. She has sinus issues and is having trouble sleeping at night. She also clenches and grinds her teeth at night while she sleeps. In the next chapter, I'll talk about what we can do for Marissa and other patients with similar issues.

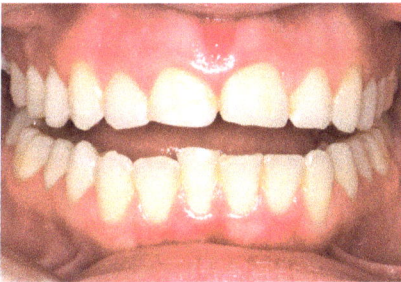 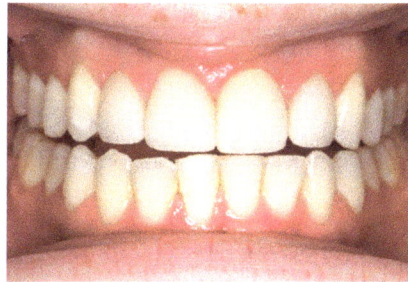

BEFORE                AFTER

See Marissa's new smile in the gallery at
**TheMillerCenter.com**.

# *Quick Quiz*

1.  Name three anatomical parts of teeth.

2.  Name one of the problems of aging teeth.

3.  Name the three components of the mouth affected by disharmony.

4.  What is parafunction?

# CHAPTER THREE

# NOSES ARE FOR BREATHING, MOUTHS ARE FOR EATING

Humans can go forty days without eating, but only three minutes without breathing. If you're not breathing well from day to day (and throughout the night), your health will decline because your body needs oxygen to survive—and thrive.

Nasal breathing is proper breathing. Breathing through your nose allows you to smell some of life's beautiful scents but this also acts as a detector when air is unhealthy—or even dangerous. The olfactory sense (sense of smell) is actually one of the strongest senses for triggering emotions and memory. How many times have you walked into a room and smelled a pleasant aroma—cookies baking or a fresh, outdoorsy scent—that reminded you of a happy time in your life?

But there is more going on with nasal breathing at the biological level. Breathing through the nose helps regulate your body temperature by cooling the pituitary gland, which helps to regulate the production of hormones in the body. It's often called the master gland because it regulates other glands that release hormones. When your nasal passages are clear, light can reach the pituitary gland, which helps to regulate sleeping patterns.[15]

The nose is also an excellent filtration system: it moisturizes the air breathed, which adds measurable amounts of liquid to your body and warms air to the optimum temperature before it reaches the lungs. The sinuses produce nitric oxide, which dilates the airway and sterilizes air breathed in by the nose, unlike mouth breathing, during which you're breathing unfiltered air.[16] Since the sinuses trap $CO_2$ when you exhale, nose breathing can promote vasodilation, which is the widening of the blood vessels.[17] $CO_2$ naturally widens the blood vessels, allowing for the release of more oxygen into the bloodstream and the body's cells, helping promote better pH balance in the body overall.[18] Balanced pH means the body is less acidic, which keeps inflammation in check. I'll talk more about the damaging effects of inflammation later in this chapter and in chapter 4.

Nose breathing keeps the passages open and, in children, helps form the sinuses, which begin growing around age four. Children who can't breathe through their noses—and so breathe through their mouths—often develop very narrow faces.[19]

Breathing through the nose promotes a more meditative state, helping you stay calmer by reducing anxiety while improving your ability to think more clearly.

When people breathe clearly through their noses, their heads are upright and in line with their spine, resulting in good balance and reduced stress to the orthopedic structures of the body. Blocked nasal

15    Lisa Bowen, "28 Reasons to Nose Breathe," Breathing Retraining Center, January 9, 2012, http://www.breathingretrainingcenter.com/blog/28-reasons-to-nose-breathe.
16    Ibid.
17    "Vasodilation–Vasoconstriction," E-Breathing.com, accessed July 18, 2018, http://www.e-breathing.com/symptoms/vasodilation.
18    Lisa Bowen, "28 Reasons to Nose Breathe," Breathing Retraining Center, January 9, 2012, http://www.breathingretrainingcenter.com/blog/28-reasons-to-nose-breathe.
19    Ibid.

passages that cause people to breathe through their mouth can lead to forward-head posture, a stooped-over position in which the head is far forward from the shoulders. The body assumes that position because it opens the airway in the throat to allow breathing to continue. In addition, every inch that the head juts forward puts an extra ten pounds of weight on the spine!

Mouth breathing can also result in inflammation of the jaw joints or TMJ for a number of reasons largely related to malfunctioning of the jaws. People breathe through their mouths because the airways through their noses are blocked. When that happens, the jaws instinctively clench during sleep to open the throat muscles and allow air in. All that clenching can stress the jaws, creating inflammation and damage to the TMJs. I'll talk more about TMJs later in the chapter.

Imagine, if you will, all the various positions and contortions the body performs as it twists to open the airway. All of those movements cause problems from your head to your toes, which explains how blocked nasal passages can actually be causing pain in your foot. I'll talk more about this in chapter 5.

## NOSE BREATHING: IMPERATIVE FOR SLEEP

Blocked nasal passages can cause sleep disordered breathing (SDB). There are three types of SDB: snoring, upper airway resistance syndrome (UARS), and obstructive sleep apnea (OSA). OSA is the most common form of SDB. The National Institutes of Health considers OSA a common disorder, affecting twelve million Americans.[20] Obstructive sleep apnea is a complete cessation of breathing during sleep for at least ten seconds. During an episode of OSA, the

---

20   Karla Diaz et al., "Obstructive Sleep Apnea Is Associated with Higher Healthcare Utilization in Elderly Patients," *Annals of Thoracic Medicine* 9, no. 2 (April–June 2014): 92–98, https://www.ncbi.nlm.nih.gov/pmc/articles/PMC4005168.

entire upper airway is blocked, causing airflow to stop and, in turn disrupts sleep because oxygen is cut off. Apnea is the collapse of the trachea. When that happens, the sleeper subconsciously—and repeatedly—awakens in an effort to breathe.

Signs and symptoms of OSA include:

- intermittent snoring;

- excessive daytime sleepiness;

- gasping for breath or choking during sleep, causing abrupt awakenings;

- nonrefreshing, fragmented sleep;

- poor memory (because the brain needs sleep to rejuvenate); and

- irritability or other personality changes.

When OSA goes untreated, it can even affect relationships: chronic snoring night after night can disrupt the sleep of partners and, ultimately, affect their health.

Left untreated, OSA can increase in severity and even lead to life-threatening illnesses such as hypertension or high blood pressure, cardiac arrhythmias or irregular heartbeats, and cerebrovascular disease, which can lead to a stroke. The link between OSA and cardiovascular issues stems largely from the reduction in oxygen levels that occurs from repeated hyperventilation (trying to breathe), the repeated disruptions in sleep, and the constant adrenaline surges that happen as the body is jarred awake to breathe, create the repeated strain to the cardiovascular system.

## RISK FACTORS OF OSA

The following are some of the factors that can put you at risk for OSA.

**Obesity**. Being overweight is one of the primary risk factors for developing OSA. According to the CDC, nearly 40 percent of adults in the US were overweight or obese in 2015–2016.[21] As obesity relates to OSA, it's something of a two-way street: being overweight can mean having a thicker neck and fatter tongue, which can lead to a narrower airway in the throat. OSA can lead to having less energy to exercise. Lack of good quality sleep can also disrupt the production of hormones that signal when it's time to eat and when it's time to stop eating. In addition, people who can't sleep often head to the fridge for a snack, thus adding calories to their day. So, while OSA is often the result of excess weight, it also compounds that very problem.

**Aging**. While OSA can affect anyone at any age, it is most common in adults aged between forty and sixty.[22] Peri and postmenopausal women may develop symptoms of OSA due to dropping hormone levels that disrupt sleep, often because of hot flashes.

**Gender**. OSA is more common in men than in women for a number of biological reasons. However, one review of current studies pointed to the discrepancy stemming from under-reporting OSA in women.[23]

**Family history**. Your chances of having OSA are higher if a family member also has, or had, it because of traits such as obesity or a

---

21  "Adult Obesity Facts," Centers for Disease Control and Prevention, accessed July 19, 2018,https://www.cdc.gov/obesity/data/adult.html.

22  "Sleep Apnea and High Blood Pressure: A Dangerous Pair," CardioSmart, American College of Cardiology, May 1, 2015, https://www.cardiosmart.org/news-and-events/2015/05/sleep-apnea-and-high-blood-pressure-a-dangerous-pair.

23  Christine Lin, Terence Davidson, and Sonia Ancoli-Israel, "Gender Differences in Obstructive Sleep Apnea and Treatment Implications," *Sleep Medicine Reviews* 12, no. 6 (December 2008): 481–496, https://www.ncbi.nlm.nih.gov/pmc/articles/PMC2642982.

recessed jaw, which tend to run in families.[24]

**Unhealthy habits**. Drinking alcohol, abusing sedatives, and smoking are unhealthy habits that can worsen sleep apnea. Alcohol and sedatives can make it more difficult to rouse from sleep, even when your breathing stops. Smoking, meanwhile, can cause irritation to the tissues of your nose and throat, further inflaming your breathing passage.[25]

**Less-than-optimum health**. Existing health problems can lead to OSA or worsen symptoms. Health issues that are associated with OSA include breathing disorders such as asthma, or hypertension, which, as I mentioned earlier, can be complicated by OSA. In fact, research has found that some 30 to 50 percent of people with high blood pressure have OSA, but it is more common in people for whom blood pressure medications have failed to help control their condition.[26]

**Anatomic abnormalities of the airway**. As I mentioned earlier, it's imperative to have open nasal passages. A blocked or inflamed nasal passage is one reason that many people suffer from OSA. Blockage anywhere in the airway, from the tip of the nose to the back of the throat behind the tongue, can also cause OSA symptoms. When you are awake, your brain signals the muscles in your airway to stiffen and allow enough air to flow through the passage. During sleep, however, the muscles of the airway relax, along with the rest of the body. Those who have OSA do not have strong enough muscles to deal with that

---

24  "Sleep Apnea: Symptoms and Risk Factors," Sleep Education, the Academy of Sleep Medicine, accessed July 19, 2018, http://www.sleepeducation.org/essentials-in-sleep/sleep-apnea/symptoms-risk-factors.

25  "Sleep Apnea," *U.S. News & World Report Health*, accessed July 19, 2018, https://health.usnews.com/health-conditions/sleep/sleep-apnea/managing.

26  "Sleep Apnea and High Blood Pressure: A Dangerous Pair," CardioSmart, American College of Cardiology, May 1, 2015, https://www.cardiosmart.org/news-and-events/2015/05/sleep-apnea-and-high-blood-pressure-a-dangerous-pair.

collapse, and so the airway closes to the point that breathing ceases.[27] In some people, a lack of collagen can decrease muscle tonus in the airway.

**Malocclusion**. When the bite is misaligned—the teeth don't come together properly—it can affect the airway and lead to sleep disturbances or OSA.

Excessive overjet, for instance, can also be a potential indicator of OSA. Overjet is a type of malocclusion (misaligned bite) in which the upper jaw extends far forward from the lower jaw. Overjet can develop in the absence of breastfeeding, as can other types of malocclusion including open bite, where there is a gap between the upper and lower teeth during a bite, and crossbite, in which a tooth or teeth either tilt in or out and therefore do not meet the tooth (or teeth) in the opposing jaw.[28]

Misaligned teeth are usually a symptom of an airway issue: if you breathe through your nose properly, you will have straight teeth, unless there are extenuating circumstances such as trauma. Breathing is the problem, not the teeth.

**Skeletal development**. How the mouth and head form during development can create risk factors for OSA.

The palate (upper arch in the mouth) of a newborn is malleable. As children develop, their tongue places pressure on their palate, which determines its shape. That happens during breastfeeding. As children learn to swallow normally, those two activities—breastfeeding and swallowing normally—enable the palate to grow to adequate height and the dental arch to form a nicely rounded, U shape, which

---

27  "What Happens during OSA," Healthy Sleep, accessed July 19, 2018, http://healthysleep. med.harvard.edu/sleep-apnea/what-is-osa/what-happens.

28  Karen Glazer Peres et al., "Exclusive Breastfeeding and Risk of Dental Malocclusion," *Pediatrics* 136, no. 1 (July 2015): e60–67,http://pediatrics.aappublications.org/content/ pediatrics/early/2015/06/09/peds.2014-3276.full.pdf.

allows the tongue to function normally.[29] If a child does not breastfeed properly, then the arch develops high and narrow, into a V shape. That shape constricts the tongue and forces it back into the airway where it blocks the flow of air, leading to OSA. A narrow, V-shaped palate can also lead to narrower nasal passages because the palate is, in fact, the floor of the nose. As the palate grows normally into a broad U-shape, the nasal passages get bigger. A V-shaped palate may mean the nasal passages are under-developed. That narrowing of the nasal passages can further constrict the flow of air.

Tongue tie may also cause jaw deformity. Tongue tie is when the tissue under the tongue is tethered to the floor of the mouth just behind the bottom teeth. That tethering can prevent the tongue from reaching the palate during formation, leading to a high, narrow, V-shaped arch.

**Inflammation**. Inflammation can stem from a number of causes and can lead to problems throughout the body, including the airways. For instance, mouth breathing can cause inflammation of the tonsils and adenoids, which can obstruct an airway. An enlarged uvula, that bit of flesh that dangles in the back of everyone's throat, can also impede airflow in the airway. When inflamed, the nasal maxillary sinuses and turbinates can also make it very difficult to breathe through your nose. Turbinates, which are portions of the nasal airway that are made of bone and soft tissue, warm and moisturize air flowing through the nose. Both the bone and tissue can enlarge and block the nasal airflow.[30] That can happen as a result of allergic responses to the environment or even to some foods. I'll talk more about inflammation and diet in the next chapter.

---

29  Brian Palmer, "The Uniqueness of the Human Airway," *Sleep Review*, March 4, 2003, http://www.sleepreviewmag.com/2003/03/the-uniqueness-of-the-human-airway.

30  Pural Goyal, "Septoplasty & Turbinate Surgery," American Rhinologic Society, accessed July 21, 2018, http://care.american-rhinologic.org/septoplasty_turbinates.

## DIAGNOSING OSA

The American Academy of Sleep Medicine (AASM) states that only a sleep physician can make the diagnosis of OSA. So while dental professionals are in a unique position to screen patients for OSA, their patients must be referred to a sleep physician for a definitive diagnosis.[31]

As a dentist, I can identify signs and symptoms that may indicate that a person has a sleep-breathing disorder. When I suspect patients may have OSA, I have them undergo a sleep study (polysomnogram, or PSG) at a sleep center. There, the patient's sleep is monitored and measured throughout the night.

The results of the sleep study look at what is known as the apnea hypopnea index (AHI), which shows the number of apneas (breathing stoppages) or hypopneas (shallow breathing) that occur during an hour of sleep. The severity of OSA is determined by the number of events per hour:[32]

- Less than 5 = no or minimal OSA

- 5 to 14 = mild OSA

- 15 to 30 = moderate

- 30 or more = severe

The study also looks at oxygen levels in the blood, which should, generally, be more than 90 percent. Depending on the study, heart rate and other measurements may be monitored in order to form a diagnosis.

---

31   T&S Therapy Centre International (La Mesa, California), "Sleep-Related Breathing Disorders and Craniofacial Pain for Adults and Children" course directed by Steven Olmos in Orlando, Florida, April 26–27, 2016.

32   "What Happens during OSA," Healthy Sleep, accessed July 19, 2018, http://healthysleep. med.harvard.edu/sleep-apnea/what-is-osa/what-happens.

# WHAT IS THE TMJ?

Airway issues can also cause problems with the TMJs.

The TMJ is a very special ball-and-socket joint, or a hinge, that is located just in front of the ear. Along with muscles and ligaments that are attached to the skull and jaws, these joints allow the mouth to open and close and the jaws to move from side to side. The TMJ also moves the lower jaw forward.

In dentistry, the abbreviation TMJ is somewhat interchangeable with TMD, which stands for temporomandibular disorder or dysfunction. TMD is a better description since it describes an internal disorder or dysfunction going on in one or both of the joints. That dysfunction is evident when there is a popping or clicking noise and/or pain when opening or closing your mouth. Upon opening, a dysfunctional set of TM joints can even lock the jaw, leaving you unable to adequately open or close your mouth. Over time, the clicks, pops, and locks in the joints can lead to joint discomfort and pain.

TMD is typically caused by an obstructed airway, which causes chronic clenching and grinding, by a trauma that dislocates the jaw or by central sensitization (CS). CS is a condition of the nervous system that is associated with the development and maintenance of chronic pain; the nervous system is in a persistent state of high reactivity or excitability, which lowers an individual's pain threshold, even after the initial injury has healed.

With today's sophisticated technologies—namely cone beam computed tomography (CBCT), CT scans, and MRIs—we can better understand the normal and dysfunctional anatomy of the temporomandibular joints. These technologies have made a significant difference in how we manage and treat temporomandibular joint disorders. The knowledge obtained from many studies that have utilized these imaging tools, combined with the information obtained from a patient's comprehensive history and examination, gives us a greater ability to interpret what may be occurring within the joints of an individual.

## TREATMENT OPTIONS

There are a variety of treatments that can begin to alleviate the problems of TMD and OSA. Which treatment is used depends on the severity of the problem and whether the patient is likely to comply with the doctor's instructions. Here are some of the options available.

### TMD Treatments

**Soft bite splint**. Short-term treatment options for TMD include a soft bite splint. Called an aqualizer, this type of appliance is worn in the mouth, similar to, but more sophisticated than, a bite guard. It's a very useful tool for temporary relief of muscle pain and joint inflammation associated with TMD. It works exceptionally well when combined with anti-inflammatories and topical muscle-relaxing creams that are also effective in joint symptom management. We give aqualizers to patients prior to fabrication of a TMD appliance.

**Laser light therapy (cold laser therapy)**. Laser light therapy can be used to provide immediate, though temporary, relief for TMD discomfort. In spite of its name, there is no heat or burning sensation with laser light therapy, which is why we refer to it in my practice as cold laser. Cold laser light therapy has been shown to increase blood circulation by stimulating the formation of additional blood vessels to replace damaged ones. New blood vessels speed up the healing process by supplying additional oxygen and nutrients needed for healing. Cold laser light therapy also stimulates the production of collagen. Collagen is the most common protein found in the body. It is the essential protein used to repair and replace damaged tissue. Cold laser light therapy also decreases swelling and reduces the excitability of inner tissue, thereby relieving pain.

**Nasal cones and sprays**. Most TMD is caused by breathing issues from inflammation or blockage in the nose. When that's the case, nasal sprays and nasal cones can help provide immediate relief.

**Appliance therapy for TMD**. All of the above therapies can be used for immediate relief prior to fabricating an oral appliance, a custom-made device made of acrylic or printed nylon and designed to be worn on the teeth. These appliances are designed to perform certain functions inside the mouth, depending on the patient's situation.

Oral appliance therapy for TMD and OSA are similar in many respects. However, if the issue is primarily TMD, patients may have to wear a night appliance and a day appliance to keep their teeth from hitting together. Every time the upper and lower teeth touch each other, the TM joint gets disturbed or compressed, causing pain to the joint tissues. Wearing separate day and night appliances allows the joints to remain undisturbed or decompressed, which allows tissue healing in the joint space. The patients are weaned off the day appliance after wearing it for twelve weeks straight, but they may continue to wear the night appliance. If the problem is primarily a breathing issue, such as mild or moderate OSA, a nighttime-only appliance may be the treatment of choice.

## OSA Treatments

Treatment options available for OSA patients include CPAP, surgery, and oral appliance therapy.

**CPAP (continuous positive airway pressure)**. With a CPAP machine, the patients wear a mask during sleep that seals over their nose and mouth, or over their nose only. The CPAP opens up their airway by feeding positive air pressure through the mask via a hose connected to the CPAP machine. CPAPs have been found effective for moderate to severe OSA, but according to the American Association for Respiratory Care, compliance with CPAP remains a challenge.[33] Its use is also associated with a number of problems, including laceration of the bridge of the nose (which is caused by the mask), rawness in the throat, bloating in the stomach, and ironically, for the patients it is designed to treat, nasal congestion and even sleep deprivation. CPAPs are also obtrusive—just ask any sleep partner of an OSA patient—and while mobile versions have been developed in recent years, they are still somewhat unwieldy and a challenge to transport.

**Surgery** is helpful where there is anatomical obstruction, such as large tonsils or adenoids, or an enlarged uvula, which I mentioned earlier. Surgery may also help nasal anatomical problems, such as the turbinate reduction and nasal valve (nostril) collapse I mentioned earlier. However, surgery has only been found to be 30 to 50 percent effective.[34]

**Oral appliance therapy for OSA**. Oral appliances are a type of treatment that the dental professional is uniquely able to provide. Oral appliance therapy for OSA is similar to that for TMD. It is noninvasive, less obtrusive than CPAP, and more effective in the treatment of mild to moderate cases of OSA. In fact, success rates have been found to be as high as 76 percent with oral appliance therapy.[35]

---

33   Dries Testelmans and Bertien Buyse, "CPAP Adherence: A Matter of Perfect Airflow Curves?" *Respiratory Care* 62, no. 4 (April 2017): 515–516.

34   T&S Therapy Centre International (La Mesa, California), "Sleep-Related Breathing Disorders and Craniofacial Pain for Adults and Children," course directed by Steven Olmos in Orlando, Florida, April 26–27, 2016.

35   Ibid.

Like the aforementioned TMD appliances, most of these are devices made of acrylic or printed nylon that fit over the teeth. They are designed to fit either one arch or both the upper and lower arches. While some boil-and-bite appliances claim to provide relief for snoring, they are not recommended because they do not specifically address the bite and TM joint relationship. Instead, OSA appliances that are custom-designed and fabricated for the individual patient can provide relief for sleep apnea. Known as mandibular repositioning appliances, these are viable solutions because they are worn during sleep and reposition the mandible (the lower jaw), advancing it forward to change the shape of the airway and open it up to make breathing easier.

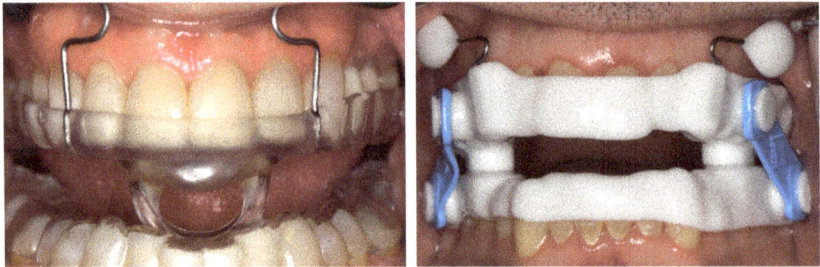

EXAMPLES OF SLEEP APNEA APPLIANCES

Patient compliance with oral appliances is significantly higher than for CPAP, reportedly at around 60 to 70 percent after three years of use.[36] Oral appliances for OSA can sometimes cause minor biting shifts that are easily corrected by removing the appliance and opening and closing the mouth a few times.

Custom-fabricated appliances are designed to treat each individual patient's problems—whether TMD, OSA, or a combination of both—following a complete assessment and comprehensive examination. That exam also shows us any other issues that need to be fixed

36    Ibid.

in a patient's mouth. In the next chapter, we'll look at some of those other issues because fixing them is the starting point for a healthier mouth and body.

# *Quick Quiz*

1. What does OSA stand for?

2. How do problems with the nose lead to or complicate OSA?

3. Name two signs/symptoms of OSA.

4. Name two treatment options for TMD.

5. Name two treatment options for OSA.

# CHAPTER FOUR

# THE FOUNDATION FOR A BEAUTIFUL SMILE

As are many patients, Eric was embarrassed by his smile. He was in his forties when he came to The Miller Center, and even though he had braces when he was younger, he was now dealing with so much wear on his upper front teeth that they were thinning and chipped. One of his upper front teeth—his upper right central incisor—was also slightly darker than the rest, potentially the result of trauma to the tooth when he was very young. During my initial consult with him, he stated that his dental "victory"—what he wanted to achieve with treatment—was for all of his front teeth to be repaired, and for them to be whiter and all the same color.

During the comprehensive dental examination, we ask patients about their history to get clues as to how the destruction in their mouth happened over time. We ask about things such as fingernail-biting habits, soda- or beer-bottle accidents, and how they chew with their misaligned teeth, all of which can help me better understand the everyday wear and tear on their teeth. Often, we find issues such as tooth mobility and sensitivity caused by that mobility, exposed dentin and cracked teeth, and myofacial pain along with difficulty in chewing.

In Eric's case, the exam determined that the amount of space between his upper and lower front teeth was constricted. That space, known as the "envelope of function," is needed to chew and is impacted during swallowing. As long as the upper and lower front teeth function within that space, or envelope, without interference from the opposing teeth, all the teeth can be protected. However, when the envelope or space is constricted, the interference from opposing teeth can be very destructive, with the most noticeable consequences being wear and chipping. While the wear and chipping on Eric's lower front teeth was minimal, there was considerable wear on the back of his upper front teeth. Every time his teeth came together during a bite or swallow, there was interference.

I talked with Eric about options to correct his constricted chewing space. To achieve this, we needed to open up his bite. That meant moving his lower front teeth back and his upper front teeth forward toward his lips. The only way to achieve those movements was with orthodontics. Had Eric opted to forgo orthodontics, his condition would have worsened to the point that he would have been untreatable.

After Eric was diagnosed and informed of his options for treatment, he decided to proceed with Invisalign clear aligner therapy. Invisalign is a series of clear plastic aligners or trays that fit perfectly over the patient's teeth. They are designed by a computer program to slowly control the movement of teeth.

# A HEALTHY MOUTH STARTS WITH A STRONG FOUNDATION

It is important to maintain good oral health in order to keep your teeth as you age. Good oral health lets you continue to chew effectively and efficiently, enjoy your food, have a pleasing appearance, be self-confident, and be free from pain and infection.[37] In fact, studies are finding that preventive dental care does improve oral health and can lower the cost of dental treatment for people who have chronic, systemic disease.[38] But regardless of the connection between the problems in the mouth and the rest of the body, good oral health is reason enough to undergo preventive dental care.

There are many variables that constitute the definition of a healthy mouth.

For one, the gum tissue (gingiva) needs to be healthy. By definition, healthy gums are pink in color, not red. They do not hurt and they don't bleed when brushed or flossed. Nor do they bleed when touched with a dental measuring device called a periodontal probe. That probe is used during a dental examination to measure from the top of the gum tissue adjacent to the tooth to the bottom of the gingival space between the gum tissue and the tooth. That gingival space is called a sulcus, as I mentioned in chapter 2. Again, a healthy sulcus measures two to three millimeters deep. Only a healthy sulcus, three millimeters or less, is a strong foundation for a healthy mouth long-term.

---

37  Bruce L. Pihlstrom et al., "Promoting Oral Health Care because of Its Possible Effect on Systemic Disease Is Premature and May Be Misleading," *Journal of the American Dental Association* 149, no. 6 (June 2018): 401–403, https://jada.ada.org/article/S0002-8177(18)30240-X/fulltext.

38  Ibid.

If the periodontal probe measures greater than three millimeters in depth, the space is no longer called the sulcus. At that point, it is referred to as a periodontal pocket. Periodontal pockets are not cleansable at home by a patient and must be treated in a dental office. Left untreated, a periodontal pocket will increase in depth, leading to periodontal disease, which can ultimately lead to the loss of the bone surrounding the teeth. That bony casing is what keeps the teeth solidly in place. That's how untreated periodontal disease can, over time, turn a healthy, solid, strong foundation into a soft, weak foundation for existing teeth and for any dental work that you may want to have done.

## THE IMPORTANCE OF BACTERIAL BALANCE

The mouth is the ideal habitat for a variety of bacteria, both good and bad. At birth, the mouth is a sterile environment. Good bacteria very quickly colonize in the mouth, beginning with the first breastfeeding. A different type of bacteria begins to colonize when the first teeth appear—a type of bacteria that thrives on a surface such as teeth. These bacteria remain in the mouth for as long as you have teeth. Other strains of bacteria that live in the mouth prefer to reside on the gums and cheeks, while bacteria that can live without oxygen tend to thrive in the crevices in the gum around the roots of the teeth.[39]

When the mouth is healthy, the normal flora (bacteria and other microorganisms) that lives there make it tougher for bad bacteria to colonize. In fact, when the flora of the mouth is healthy, the good bacteria feed off the nutrients there. In turn, they help synthesize the

39   Kenneth Todar, "The Normal Bacterial Flora of Humans," *Todar's Online Textbook of Bacteriology*, accessed July 22, 2018, http://textbookofbacteriology.net/normalflora_3.html.

vitamins in your body, which can improve your body's immune system.[40]

Unfortunately, oral florae are also at the root of problems in the mouth, including abscesses and gum disease. If they're allowed to build up, they can begin to break down the gum tissue, leading to periodontal disease. If they get into the deeper tissues of the body, they can cause infections at the systemic level.[41]

That's why it is key to maintain bacterial balance in the mouth by keeping teeth clean. That allows good bacteria to thrive and helps keep bad bacteria at bay.

## THE DETRIMENTAL EFFECTS OF SUGAR

Sugar is toxic. Period. As a dentist, of course I'm interested in sugar from the aspect of how it can cause decay in teeth. Too much sugar can upset the bacterial balance in your mouth; the bacteria in your mouth feed on sugar, and the by-products they release in the process can lead to tooth demineralization. But as I mentioned in the introduction, I'm a hybrid dentist: I'm curious about all aspects of creating good dental health in my patients. Therefore, the rest of this chapter is devoted to helping you understand some of the other aspects of good health.

Nothing good comes from sugar ingestion. I found out for myself the detrimental effects of sugar on the body. For thirty-some years, my blood pressure was always around 130/90. But six months after changing my diet to one with far less sugar and fewer carbs, it has dropped to around 120/80—a much healthier reading. I don't exercise as much as I used to, so I can absolutely point to the change in my diet as the reason for my lowered blood pressure.

Sugar produces an immediate effect on the immune system. Even sugar substitutes such as Equal and NutraSweet contain aspartame,

---

40   Ibid.
41   Ibid.

which is known to metabolize to 10 percent methanol—something you don't want in your body. Stevia, however, is a safe sugar substitute.

Other reasons to avoid sugar include:

- **Weight gain**. Fructose is one type of simple sugar, and the sodas and fruit juices that people consume daily are loaded with the stuff. Sugary drinks are little more than liquid calories—a 16-ounce soda has 52 grams of sugar, which is more than 10 percent of daily intake for a 2,000-calorie diet.[42] Research has found that children and adults who consume sugar-sweetened beverages weigh more, on average.[43]

- **Increased risk of chronic disease**. High-sugar diets have been linked to obesity, inflammation, stroke-causing levels of triglycerides, and elevated blood sugar and blood pressure levels. One study found that people who consumed nearly one-fifth of their calories from sugar had more than a 35 percent greater risk of dying from heart disease than people whose calorie intake was only 8 percent from added sugar.[44] Prolonged consumption of high quantities of sugar in a diet can lead to insulin resistance, which can create an imbalance in the production of insulin in the body and increase the risk of diabetes. Diabetes is a disease in which the pancreas does not secrete insulin as needed to regulate blood glucose

---

42   Jillian Kubala, "11 Reasons Why Too Much Sugar Is Bad for You," Healthline, June 3, 2018, https://www.healthline.com/nutrition/too-much-sugar.

43   V. S. Malik et al., "Sugar-Sweetened Beverages and Weight Gain in Children and Adults: A Systematic Review and Meta-Analysis," *The American Journal of Clinical Nutrition* 98, no. 4 (October 2013): 1084–1102, https://www.ncbi.nlm.nih.gov/pubmed/23966427.

44   Q. Yang et al., "Added Sugar Intake and Cardiovascular Diseases Mortality among US Adults," *Journal of the American Medical Association Internal Medicine* 174, no. 4 (April 2014): 516–524, https://www.ncbi.nlm.nih.gov/pubmed/24493081.

levels. One study that looked at people from more than 175 countries found a 1.1 percent higher risk of developing diabetes for every 150 calories of sugar consumed daily—roughly one can of soda.[45]

- **Accelerates aging**. Studies have shown that consuming high quantities of sugar has been shown to increase aging at the cellular level.[46] Sugar can react with proteins in your body to produce advanced glycation end products (AGEs), which damage collagen and elastin. Collagen and elastin are the proteins that help the skin have a youthful appearance; damaging them can prematurely age the skin.[47]

- **Saps energy**. Although people often reach for something sugary when they need a boost of energy, sugar spikes the levels of blood sugar and insulin in your body. Yes, that tends to temporarily increase your energy level. However, foods loaded with processed sugar, without also having protein, fiber, or fat, can cause you to crash following the sugar high.[48]

- **Increased inflammation**. Sugar creates a lot of inflammation in the body, and when the muscles, joints, and nerves are inflamed, they can be the source of a lot of pain. Inflammation combined with obesity can raise your risk of cancer

45   Basu Sanjay et al., "The Relationship of Sugar to Population-Level Diabetes Prevalence: An Econometric Analysis of Repeated Cross-Sectional Data," *PLoS One* 8, no. 2 (2013): e57873, https://www.ncbi.nlm.nih.gov/pmc/articles/PMC3584048.

46   Ibid.

47   Jillian Kubala, "11 Reasons Why Too Much Sugar Is Bad For You," Healthline, June 3, 2018, accessed July 22, 2018, https://www.healthline.com/nutrition/too-much-sugar.

48   Ibid.

of the esophagus and small intestine.[49] High fructose intake has also been linked to increased risk of kidney disease, fatty liver disease, and dementia.[50]

## *Signs of inflammation include*[51]

- chronic aches and pains including headaches, neck pain, and muscle or joint soreness;

- propensity for illness;

- difficulty losing weight and a "spare tire" around the midsection;

- lack of exercise;

- lack of energy; and

- lack of skin tone.

Lowering inflammation—and pain levels—means switching up your diet to avoid inflammatory foods. A healthy diet allows your body to decrease inflammation and heal with optimum success during therapy for OSA. The key is to begin changing your diet to lower inflammation a little at a time, until you find out what works for you. For instance, while coffee is sometimes among those items listed as inflammatory, other studies have found coffee to be an antioxidant that can reduce the risk of cancer. I still drink coffee, but instead of milk or half-and-half, which I find to be inflammatory, I use almond milk. Why almond over soy milk? Simply because I

---

49   Natasa Tasevska et al., "Sugars in Diet and Risk of Cancer in the NIH-AARP Diet and Health Study," *International Journal of Cancer* 130, no. 1 (January 2012): 159–169, https://www.ncbi.nlm.nih.gov/pmc/articles/PMC3494407.

50   Jillian Kubala, "11 Reasons Why Too Much Sugar Is Bad For You," Healthline, June 3, 2018, https://www.healthline.com/nutrition/too-much-sugar.

51   "The DeFlaming Guidelines," Ormond Beach, Florida: DeFlame Enterprises, 2009.

prefer the taste, not because soy bothers me, as it does some people. Here are some guidelines for what to eat—and not to eat—that work for many people:

- **Vegetables**. Eat more green, leafy vegetables, which contain folic acid and a coenzyme to aid in balancing metabolism. Also eat plenty of other vegetables daily for a healthy dose of vitamins.

- **Fresh fruits**. Fresh fruit blended into smoothies with protein powder supplements provide an excellent source of vitamin and mineral nutrients along with a portion of daily protein needs. I make a morning fruit shake almost daily. I simply blend fresh or frozen fruit with a scoop of protein powder and almond milk. It's a refreshing and filling way to start my day.

- **Fish** provides daily protein and essential fatty acids, which assist in digestion.

- **Free-range eggs and poultry**. Eat more free-range eggs and poultry—avoid red meat and grain-fed eggs and poultry since these contain steroids that reduce the immune system's ability to heal, and arachidonic acid that can cause vascular and neuropathic pain due to inflammation.

- **Soy and almond products** should be substituted for dairy products, and then only in condiment-sized portions. While calcium is important, milk and cheese products contain phosphates that acidify in the blood, which can predispose you to pain. (Citracal, an over-the-counter supplement, is the best form of calcium to take.) Choose butter instead of margarine—margarine contains hydrogenated oil, which cannot be digested.

- **Unleavened bread** may be preferable, especially for people who get migraines from ingesting yeast.

- **Drink plenty of water** every day—at least six to eight glasses—to flush your system. A good rule of thumb to follow for daily water consumption is to divide your weight (in pounds) by two. The result is the number of ounces of water you should drink each day. [52]

Occasionally, herbal teas may also be consumed, but avoid cola and caffeine products because these can increase the acidic pH of your blood.

Why does blood pH matter? Because low blood pH means your blood is acidic, and acidic blood is low in oxygen. When you don't have enough oxygen in your blood, your body's ability to heal itself is diminished. By eating foods that are alkaline and low acid, and then taking the right supplements, you can neutralize your blood pH. That's why veggies and protein are good for you—they help neutralize your blood pH—while sugar and carbs, wheat, caffeine, carbonated drinks, and so on can raise your blood acid.

Acidic blood is usually found in people who are addicted to carbs. They crave starchy foods because they have too much yeast in their gut. That can result in a condition known as "leaky gut." Leaky gut occurs when there is such an overgrowth of candida yeast in the gut that it causes tiny holes to form in the wall of the gut. When that happens, harmful microorganisms are able to literally "leak" through the bowel walls and get into the circulatory system. Instead of good nutrients getting into your bloodstream to nourish you and give you vitality, those harmful microorganisms can trigger the immune

---

52  T&S Therapy Centre International (La Mesa, California), "Sleep-Related Breathing Disorders and Craniofacial Pain for Adults and Children."

system, which can wreak all kinds of havoc on the body: inflammation, food allergies, arthritis, eczema, and worse.[53]

## TREATMENTS, SUPPLEMENTS, AND SELF-CARE

Proper nutrition is crucial for healthy dentition and oral tissues. But many people are deficient in the nutrients that keep the mouth and body healthy. In particular, deficiencies in folate, calcium, fluoride, and vitamins A, B, C, and D can affect the oral cavity and lead to decay and other problems.[54]

Treatments, supplements, and self-care can improve your oral health and overall health. In fact, when I first began offering whitening, I wanted to know whether I could help with the patient's health and healing at the same time. At one point, I considered bringing the "ideal" all-natural toothpaste to market. It would consist of the following supplements: fluoride, coenzyme Q10, and proteolytic enzymes.

Here are some of the benefits of supplements, along with a few tips for better self-care at home.

**Calcium and vitamin D**. Bone mass in the oral cavity develops during childhood but reaches its peak in early adulthood. After that, the body begins to lose bone mass in the mouth and overall. Calcium is essential for strong bones, blood clotting, and healthy nerves and muscles. Calcium and vitamin D go hand-in-hand because vitamin D helps the body absorb calcium—and phosphorus—from the food you

---

53  "Candida Yeast Infection, Leaky Gut, Irritable Bowel, and Food Allergies," National Candida Center, accessed July 29, 2018, https://www.nationalcandidacenter.com/Leaky-Gut-and-Candida-Yeast-Infection-s/1823.htm.

54  Matthew Pflipsen and Yevgeniy Zenchenko, "Nutrition for Oral Health and Oral Manifestations of Poor Nutrition and Unhealthy Habits," *General Dentistry* 6, no. 6 (November/December 2017):36–43.

eat.[55] Studies have found that people who take calcium supplements have less bone loss and fewer fractures, and that vitamin D supplements are most effective when combined with calcium supplements.[56] Studies also found that having adequate amounts of calcium and vitamin D can help combat periodontal disease by keeping inflammation in check.[57]

**Fluoride**. Caries (cavities) are one of the greatest risks to permanent teeth. Early treatment with fluoride is key to prevention. That includes using toothpaste with fluoride as soon as teeth begin to emerge. However, with aging, even healthy gums can slowly recede and leave the cementum or hard covering over the root of the tooth exposed. Since that area of the tooth is closer to the nerve, greater sensitivity to cold can develop. To combat the problem, dentists often prescribe a higher concentration of fluoride toothpaste. Why? Fluoride is a sensitivity stop-gap. On a microscopic level, dentin and cementum are made up of tubules that run from near the nerve to the exterior of the tooth. When you drink a cold beverage, the cold passes through the tubules and goes directly to the nerve area. Fluoride ions block the tubules to prevent pain. However, blocked tubules hinder the ability to whiten the teeth. Fluoride, however, is a great desensitizer after teeth whitening.

We strongly suggest topical fluoride for all our patients after their teeth are cleaned because it creates a shield against bacteria that can break down tooth structure. Most of our patients have the optional treatment in-house after a cleaning. I also suggest over-the-counter or prescription fluoride for patients who are very susceptible to decay.

---

55    Robert P. Heaney, "Vitamin D: Role in the Calcium and Phosphorus Economies," chap. 34 in *Vitamin D*, 3rd ed., ed. David Feldman, J. Wesley Pike, and John S. Adams (London: Academic Press, 2011): 607–624.

56    Charles Hildebolt et al., "Calcium and Vitamin D Use among Adults in Periodontal-Disease Maintenance Programs," *British Dental Journal* 206, no. 12 (November 29, 2012): 627–617.

57    Ibid.

**Coenzyme Q10** is an anti-inflammatory that helps heal gum tissue. Each cell in your body has an "engine" known as the mitochondria. Coenzyme Q10 boosts that cell engine to help with cell healing, which leads to tissue healing. CoQ10 is found in foods such as broccoli, spinach, mackerel, and sardines.

**Vitamin C**. The main role of vitamin C is to manufacture collagen, a protein that forms the basis of connective tissue, which is the most abundant tissue in the body and acts as a cementing substance between cells. Vitamin C is also critical to immune and antiviral functions in the body because it has a role in the production of antibodies and in the function of inflammation-fighting white blood cells. It helps the nervous system function, protects the body against damage by free radicals and the effects of aging, and helps lower the risk of cancer and heart disease.[58]

Collagen is the primary protein component of teeth and bones.[59] In fact, collagen, along with vitamin C, comprises the structures of the teeth and mouth including the dentin, pulp, cementum, periodontal fibers, connective tissues, muscles, nerves, periodontal ligaments, and tendons.[60] Although not as common in developed countries, very low levels of vitamin C in the diet can lead to scurvy, which is first seen in the breakdown of the gums. A diet rich in fruits and vegetables can provide healthy doses of vitamin C.

**Enzymes**. Unlike commercially sold toothpastes, which contain abrasives such as silica to break down plaque, I would add a proteolytic

58  Rachel Hall, "Vitamin C," Evolve Dental Healing, August 12, 2016, accessed July 23, 2018, https://evolvedental.com.au/vitamin-c.
59  Matthew Pflipsen and Yevgeniy Zenchenko, "Nutrition for Oral Health and Oral Manifestations of Poor Nutrition and Unhealthy Habits," *General Dentistry* 6, no. 6 (November/December 2017):36–43.
60  Ibid.

enzyme called papain to my toothpaste because it breaks down plaque naturally and safely without damaging teeth. Digestive enzymes can help prevent cavities and gum disease when used topically and as supplemental treatments.

As I mentioned earlier in the chapter, periodontal diseases result when microbes colonize and grow on teeth and tissues in the mouth. That's caused when oral flora grows as a result of food debris that is trapped and left in between teeth and other areas in the mouth. That flora produces acids that lead to tooth decay and gum injury. Oral enzymes help control flora because they break down the food debris, eliminating the nutrition that bad bacteria feed on. Saliva can then wash away the bacteria, deterring or preventing decay and disease. Enzymes also help heal mouth sores, which can serve as openings for bad bacteria to enter the body and cause infection.[61]

**Brushing and flossing**. Of course, the best way to give the mouth a fighting chance against decay is with regular brushing and flossing. I recommend brushing at least twice a day for about one minute each time and then flossing. I also strongly suggest flossing right before going to bed because you don't want food particles hanging out in between your teeth all night while you're sleeping. Again, left on the teeth, food can fester and cause cavities.

When flossing, wrap the floss around the neck of each tooth to create the letter C, and then floss up the tooth and into the gum line. The goal is to remove debris between the teeth and under the gum line. Holding the floss too taut when passing it between the teeth can prevent you from getting at the debris under the gums between each tooth and can even damage the gum tissue between the teeth (the papilla).

While brushing and flossing are the basics for keeping your mouth

---

61   "Preventing Periodontal Disease: Brushing, Flossing, Enzymes," Enzyme Essentials, accessed July 24, 2018, https://www.enzymeessentials.com/HTML/dental.html.

and teeth strong and healthy, as you can, undoubtedly, now see, there is a whole lot more to consider when a problem becomes apparent. But the reward is a happy, healthy mouth and a healthy body overall.

## ERIC'S "VICTORY"

Eric went through one year of treatment wearing Invisalign, changing out the aligners as prescribed. He wore the aligners for a year, which changed his bite so that there was no interference. "It was something that I never really noticed until I had completed the Invisalign, and then I actually could feel that I was no longer banging into these teeth," he said after the treatment. We had achieved what Eric needed for long-term success: ideally aligned teeth and plenty of room for his front teeth to function during all mouth movements.

Eric also had four veneers applied to his front four teeth. "I'll admit I was a little nervous to get these veneers," he said. "I wanted a really natural look. ... But once they were done, they were tremendous. I look at the teeth and you can't tell that they are not my actual teeth. ... And I asked my wife and she said, 'You just look like you have excellent teeth.'"

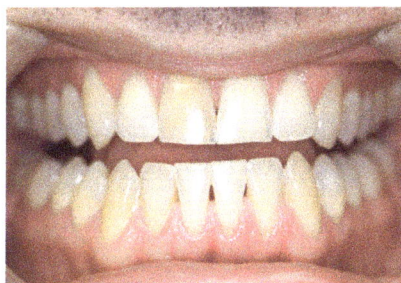 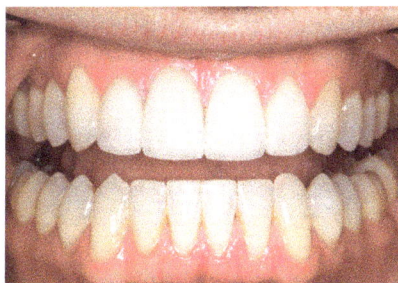

BEFORE                    AFTER

Eric's testimonial can be viewed at
**www.TheMillerCenter.com**.

# *Quick Quiz*

1. What is the sulcus?

2. Name three ways sugar is detrimental to your health.

3. What is the main role of vitamin C in the body?

4. How do enzymes help improve oral health?

5. How does fluoride protect teeth?

# CHAPTER FIVE

# ACHIEVING ESTHETIC EXCELLENCE THROUGH DENTAL RESTORATION

D an has been a patient of mine for years. Over time, he and I talked about treatment to align his bite because his upper and lower teeth did not come together in a stable way. But for many years, he chose not to undergo any of the treatments I suggested.

When Dan finally decided to have some work done, he came to me to discuss cosmetic options for his upper front teeth. His teeth appeared small, and when he smiled, they barely showed.

During my examination of Dan, which included discussing his health history, I found out that he had been diagnosed a few years earlier with spinal stenosis in his lumbar region (lower back). Stenosis refers to the abnormal narrowing of the bone channel in the spine, which houses the spinal nerves (spinal cord). In lumbar stenosis, the spinal nerves become compressed and can produce symptoms of sciatica, which is tingling, weakness, numbness, or pain that radiates from the lower back and into the buttocks and legs, especially with activity. He had undergone back surgery for the condition, but was still experiencing pain in his back.

Dan also had trouble sleeping—he woke up four to five times a night—and his wife reported that he snored loudly. Snoring is a sign that the sleeper is trying to breathe through a small airway.

It took a little digging to figure out what was causing Dan's issues. To find out where his primary pathology was, I felt his jaw joints to see if there was any clicking or popping when he moved his mouth. Feeling that there were likely some issues with his TM joint, I inserted two tongue depressors in his mouth, one on each side, to decompress his TM joint. Not only did he immediately feel better, he was able to stand upright. That indicated to me that an issue with his TM joints might be the primary reason for the pain in his lower back.

To help confirm my suspicions, I also took a scan of his TM joints, using a cone beam computed tomography (CBCT) machine. After those tests, I still thought that there was something going on anatomically, so I conducted motor nerve reflex testing (MNRT) to see if the TM joints were the primary cause of his pathology. The results of the MNRT did, in fact, support my theory that TMD was directly affecting his back.

Motor nerve reflex testing is a series of tests of neurological reflexes developed by Dr. John Beck, an orthopedic surgeon. They provide a neuromuscular way to evaluate posture. We humans stand erect. That has many advantages in the human world, but with that vertical orientation comes some major liabilities. If our brains stopped telling our muscles what to do, we would fall over because we are inherently unstable. Standing up against gravity is a big job. We expend far more calories on antigravity work than anything else we do. Running a twenty-six-mile marathon only adds 30 percent to the calories we would burn anyway just standing up. Maintaining posture exposes the body to a greater amount of wear and tear. This is why efficiency is such a big deal when it comes to posture. Normal posture protects the body from injury and conserves energy.

Posture is dynamic; it has to be. It's about being in the best position at the right time. Our brain has to know where to put us in that best position during all of our different movements. But nerve injury will throw off ideal posture. Injury to a nerve creates inflammation (neuritis). Inflamed nerves create misinformation to the brain, which in turn throws off the posture.

Dr. Beck explained that having bad posture is like having a powerful sports car that has dirty spark plugs. It may look good, but it's not running up to its full potential. Its timing is off and it needs a tune-up. MNRT helps to identify areas of postural injuries so they can be corrected. Since posture is guided by involuntary reflexes coming out of the brain and central nervous system, testing the reflexes using MNRT to measure weaknesses and strengths in the muscles lets us know what the reflexes are up to.

MNRT is part of the initial, comprehensive patient examination at my practice. That initial exam screens for a variety of dental and/ or medical issues with each patient. It involves a system of screening for head pain, jaw joint dysfunction, airway obstruction, tooth decay, gum disease, and how the upper and lower teeth come together. It's very all-inclusive.

I like to gather all of the patient's data in our first appointment. Conversation with patients during their initial examination includes the discussion of their chief complaint and what they would consider to be their big "victory," or the primary goal they hope to accomplish with treatment. The use of the term *victory* in describing the patient's goal is the inspiration of Dr. Daniel Klauer, one of my mentors and a leader in the field of dental solutions for TMD and sleep disordered breathing. The approach in that initial exam fully utilizes the knowledge and skill that dentistry has to offer health care.

While the initial exam is comprehensive, sometimes a second visit of fact finding is needed. At that time, we may take more photographs of the patient's smile or more close-up photos of the patient's teeth. Teeth close-ups may also include putty models, or impressions of the upper and lower jaws that are poured in plaster or stone. These models provide a very up-close look at how the patient's teeth are aligned, come together, and function together. X-rays, of course, are an important part of the dental fact finding. The CBCT 3-D x-ray aids not only in dental diagnosis but can also be important when evaluating jaw joint dysfunction and possible airway obstruction, which can lead to sleep disturbances.

The comprehensive evaluation is important because it helps us see how, for example, patients may be having pain in their foot that's actually coming from their TM joint. My dental assistant has had a history of discomfort in his left shoulder. Through our comprehensive examination process, we were able to determine that his shoulder pain was caused primarily by an issue in his right foot. To resolve the problem, he now wears a small silicone separator between his big toe and index toe on his right foot. He wears the separator inside his shoes; as soon as he places it between his toes, his shoulder pain goes away.

In my evaluation of my patient Dan, I determined that the primary reason for the pain in his lower back, and the reason for his snoring and sleep disturbances, was likely an issue with his TM joints.

His treatment began with wearing oral appliances day and night for twelve weeks, after which he would be weaned off the daytime appliance. However, he would continue to wear the nighttime appliance long-term to address his sleep disorder. These treatments would help restore some of the function to Dan's mouth before we addressed the cosmetic aspect of his upper front teeth.

# RESTORATIVE VERSUS COSMETIC DENTISTRY

In my practice, we address patients' issues through two avenues of dentistry: restorative and cosmetic.

Restorative dentistry refers to replacing missing teeth or parts of the tooth structure, including fillings, or repairing damage that may be due to decay, deterioration, or the fracture of a tooth. Examples of restorations include fillings, crowns, bridges, implants, and dentures. I'll talk more about these in the next chapter.

Cosmetic dentistry is one aspect of restorative dentistry. Cosmetic dentistry generally refers to any dental procedures that improve the appearance of the teeth and gums. It primarily focuses on the improvement of esthetics and color; teeth position, shape, and size; and overall smile appearance.

Porcelain veneers, bonding and teeth whitening fall under the cosmetic dentistry umbrella, but no restorative dentistry is involved in whitening teeth. I'll discuss these and other cosmetic procedures in chapter 7.

Dental health issues such as decay or gum disease must be addressed before moving ahead with cosmetic dental treatments. However, restorative dentistry is often used as a means to an end in cosmetic dentistry. For instance, we can make crowns very esthetic, beautiful, and natural looking.

With so much at stake with either of these areas of dentistry—restorative or cosmetic—it's vitally important to understand everything that is going on in the mouth before any work is done. That's why the comprehensive exam looks not only at the problems existing in the mouth today but also what led to the problems so that they can be addressed as part of any dental care.

## THE SMILE ANALYSIS

You may have heard the term *smile analysis* used in dentistry. It's actually a very subjective term because there are no set-in-stone guidelines; all dentists have their own version of what it means to analyze a smile.

Basically, a smile analysis is about collecting data to help determine exactly what the patient is looking for in a smile. No matter what else we find upon examination, patients want treatment that ensures a smile that functions well and is pleasing to look at.

My smile analysis begins with a questionnaire to help me better understand what the patients don't like about their existing smiles and what they want their smiles to look like. Questions we ask may include:

- Are any of your teeth yellow, stained, or somewhat discolored?

- Would you like your teeth to be whiter?

- Do you have any gaps or spaces between your teeth?

- Are any of your teeth turned, crooked, or uneven?

- Are you missing any teeth?

- Do you see any pitting or defects on the surfaces of your teeth?

- Are the edges of any teeth worn down, chipped, or uneven?

- Do any of your teeth appear too small, short, large, or long?

- Do you have any prior dental work that appears "unnatural?"

- Do you have any crowns or bridges that appear dark at the edge of your gum lines?

- Do you have any gray, black, gold, or silver (mercury) fillings in your teeth?

- Do you have a "gummy" smile; does too much of your gums show when smiling?

- Are your gums red, sore, puffy, bleeding, or receded?

- Does the appearance of your smile inhibit you from laughing or smiling?

- When being photographed, do you smile with your lips closed instead of flashing a full smile?

- Are you self-conscious about your teeth or smile?

- Are you interested in Botox and/or dermal fillers?

My smile analysis also involves taking a series of photographs of the patient's existing situation. These pictures include the smile and teeth from different angles. First, I take a picture of a full-face smile. I do that for two reasons: one is simply for the patient records, but the other reason is that I want to see what the patients' smile looks like as it relates to their face. From there, I zoom in to capture just the patients' smile from the front and from both sides. That's followed by a series of photographs with the patients' cheeks retracted, views that show more of the teeth and gums. The last two photographs of the smile analysis series are of the biting surfaces of upper and lower dental teeth arches.

The last piece of the overall smile analysis exam is the taking of study models. These are, essentially, casts of the teeth and mouth. I take two sets. The first is the "before" set. After these are taken, I don't touch them. The "before" model is a great way to show the patients what *all of their teeth* look like at that time: before treatment. I use the second set to create the patients' vision of what they would like their teeth to look like. This second set is a diagnostic-wax up. I use white material that looks like teeth to form beautiful mock-ups so that the patients have a very clear understanding of what their new smile will look like. The diagnostic wax-up becomes the blueprint of the patient's new smile.

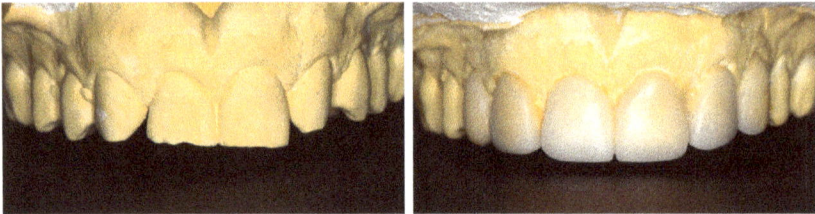

BEFORE                                    AFTER

There are a lot of computer-generated software programs available today that show before-and-after images, potentially projecting the results. I have owned and used top-of-the-line, computer-generated smile design software in the past. However, I find that using the wax-on-stone models is much more accurate.

Again, a smile analysis can be very subjective. Some dentists think a smile analysis is just a before-and-after, computer-generated smile design. Some dentists simply ask a few questions and then tell the patients what they need. But a thorough esthetic dentist asks questions, takes photographs, shows the patients what their smile could look like, and listens to the patients as they express their desires. I don't tell them what they need; I educate the patients, listen to what they want in a smile, and show them the wax-up of their smile. All that is left is for the patients to say yes to my recommendations.

# THE SMILE MAKEOVER

Some patients have so much going on in their mouth that to end with the best esthetic result, they undergo a smile makeover. With a smile makeover, you can transform your smile and your entire appearance.

Some of the problems a smile makeover may address include the following:

- **Yellowed or stained teeth.** Some foods cause discolorations. Discolored teeth look more aged than youthful teeth, which are bright and white yet look natural.

- **Chipped or broken teeth.** Damaged teeth create disharmony in the mouth and take away from a nice smile.[62]

- **Fractured teeth.** Fractures are not only painful, but make teeth unstable. They can and should be repaired as part of restoration before cosmetic procedures.

- **Irregularly shaped or disproportionate teeth**. Teeth have an ideal proportion, specific to each patient. A pleasant smile is generally defined as one that has two dominant front teeth and a four-to-five width-to-length ratio, which also guides the dimensions of the other front teeth, creating a balanced smile line.[63]

- **Short or small teeth.** The smile appears less youthful when the teeth are short, which can impact the appearance of the face overall. Long, square teeth can, for instance, slim a round face.[64]

---

62  "Smile Makeover: Reinvent Your Smile," Consumer Guide to Dentistry, accessed July 27, 2018, https://www.yourdentistryguide.com/smile-makeover.

63  Ibid.

64  Ibid.

- **Tooth texture.** This can distract from an otherwise pleasing smile, but crowns and veneers can be made to have the most natural-looking appearance for the patient's face.

- **Inconsistent spacing, or overlapped, or gapped teeth**. These can be difficult to clean and usually create a less-than-ideal smile.

- **Missing teeth.** Gaps in rows of teeth are not only unattractive but can affect your bite and even promote tooth decay.

- **An uneven gum line.** An asymmetrical gum line is another distracting—and aging—feature, but it can be modified to create symmetry.

- **A gummy smile.** Too much gum can make teeth appear shorter and more aged. Again, longer teeth make for a more youthful smile.

A smile makeover typically involves one or more restorative and/or cosmetic procedures, each customized to the individual's needs and wants. A smile makeover can involve a combination of several treatments (I'll talk more about these treatments in chapter 7):

- Teeth whitening to eliminate dental stains.

- Porcelain veneers, which are porcelain shells that can conceal cosmetic imperfections.

- Dental bonding, an efficient, cost-effective alternative to porcelain veneers that involves molding composite resin over the teeth to improve their appearance.

- Laser gum contouring to correct extended or imbalanced gum lines by removing excess tissue

- Clear aligners to gradually straighten the teeth.

- Botox cosmetic and dermal fillers to smooth wrinkles, add skin volume, and provide a powerful complement to your smile.

During the consultation for a smile makeover, I perform a full examination of your smile. I look at your smile line, or the curvature of your top front teeth, which should follow the same curvature as your bottom lip when you smile. I also look at factors such as the color, shape, width and length, and angle of your teeth; the health and shape of your gums; the shape of your lips and the underlying support structures; and even facial features such as your skin tone.

As with all patient cases, I also evaluate your oral health, and we have an in-depth conversation about what you wish to achieve with a smile makeover.

To help you understand what to expect from a smile makeover, I can also show you before-and-after photos of my patients who have undergone the various treatments at our practice. Once we determine treatment options, then I create the diagnostic wax-ups that I discussed earlier. With those wax-ups, you have the opportunity to provide me with feedback to help me create the smile you desire and deserve.

## MAKING THE MOUTH HEALTHY WITH GUM GRAFTING

As I mentioned earlier, the mouth must be healthy before cosmetic procedures can begin. Sometimes that involves more extensive procedures, as was the case with Melody. She was in her midfifties when she came in for a visit. The problem was that she hated dental work. I literally had to beg her to protect her cracked teeth with crowns. And she had one tooth that desperately needed a gum graft.

However, Melody alternated her cleanings with my office with visits to a periodontist's office. A periodontist specializes in gum tissue. In spite of my assessment that she needed gum grafting, she claimed her periodontist insisted that the area in question was stable. But to me, the area was far from stable. Her gum tissue was bright red and bled upon probing, something healthy gum tissue does not do. It was also very sensitive to touch. That's because there was also recession showing on her front tooth—a lot of her tooth root was exposed. In fact, there was so much erosion on the tooth that I could see the nerve beginning to show through the root surface. Clefting was also appearing in her gum tissue. Clefting starts at the gum line by a tooth and is shaped like a small V in the gum tissue. If not treated, the small V turns into a long, wider V and then the gum tissue proceeds to open up at that spot like a zipper. I told Melody that she could be in denial that a problem existed. Eventually, she would lose the tooth if she didn't treat it with a gum graft, which would alleviate the clefting, cover up the root surface, and repair the gum recession.

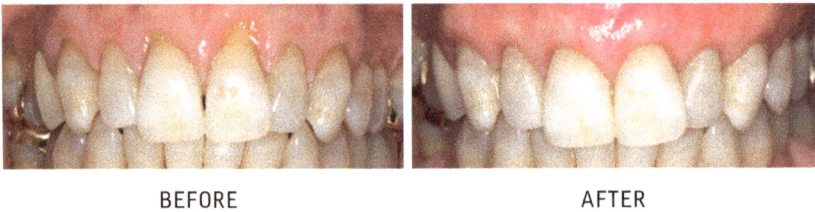

BEFORE                                    AFTER

Healthy gum tissue protects your teeth from periodontal disease and sensitivity while giving you a great smile. Aggressive tooth brushing and clefting, which is a form of periodontal disease, are two primary causes of recession. Plaque accumulates more in the clefting V shape of the gum tissue, and that plaque buildup can put you at risk for gum recession, tooth root sensitivity, loss of supporting bone, tooth decay, and eventually, tooth loss—in short, an unattractive smile.[65]

---

65  "Gum Grafting," BioHorizons, accessed July 28, 2018, http://www.biohorizons.com/gumgrafting-benefits.aspx.

Gum recession is commonly treated with a grafting procedure that involves taking gum tissue from the palate, or the roof of the mouth, creating unnecessary pain and discomfort.[66] In my office, we no longer take gum tissue from the palate. I routinely do gum grafting with an allograft material, usually one called AlloDerm. An allograft is donated tissue that has been processed to remove all cells. There's no DNA, no blood associated with this product. It is used as a gum matrix or scaffold that helps the patient's own tissue to be placed almost where the gum tissue started when it was healthy.

Allografting is an excellent safety profile and a predictable alternative to your own tissue. The esthetics are exceptional. After the tissue heals, you can't even tell that gum surgery was performed. Sometimes when your own tissue is used from the palate to repair the gum, there is a little lump of tissue by the tooth where the gum graft was placed. There may also be a slightly different color of gum tissue in the area. That doesn't happen with an allograft, specifically with AlloDerm.

Again, taking gum tissue from the palate can be quite painful for a few days after the surgery. It can be painful in two places: the palate where the tissue was taken, and the gum area by the tooth that was being treated. With allografting, there is little to no pain, just some mild soreness. There is also less potential for complications with an allograft than there is when dealing with tissue from the palate.

Melody recently got her gum graft done by her periodontist. Even though she did not have me perform her gum surgery, I was ecstatic that she had finally gotten it done! I had explained the importance of this grafting procedure to her for the past few years, but the patient and her periodontist didn't think her gum problem was serious enough to warrant surgery. The fact that her periodontist *finally* performed this surgery meant that Melody's tooth was healthier than it had been

---

66    Ibid.

for a very long time, and that her tooth's long-term prognosis became so much better: she will have this tooth in her mouth for longer than she would have if she had continued to put the graft off. Had Melody and her periodontist performed this gum graft sooner, might she have given this tooth an even longer life expectancy? We'll never know. It's so important to be proactive.

## TMJ AND OPEN AIRWAY—COMPONENTS OF A HEALTHY MOUTH

When considering all the components of a healthy mouth, we sometimes have to address TM joints and/or sleep disorders, as was the case with Dan, who was in his early forties.

Reece was only twenty-one when he came into my office wanting to have a broken tooth fixed. That was his chief "victory": to see that tooth repaired.

Through my comprehensive examination of Reece, I found that not only was his upper right, first premolar broken, but there were other teeth in his mouth that were broken and worn down. Why, you might ask, did a twenty-one-year-old have so much tooth deterioration or destruction? During the exam, I noted that Reece had a long history of snoring and grinding his teeth while he slept.

Unfortunately, we weren't able to save the tooth in question—disappointing news for Reece and his mom, who brought him to that first appointment. Instead, the tooth needed to be extracted and the solution for replacing it was with a dental implant. (See chapter 6 for more information about implants.)

But I also explained to Reece and his mom that restoring that one tooth was not the long-term answer for his dental issues. His snoring and broken/worn down teeth indicated that he was having trouble breathing at night, which meant his airway from his nose to his throat needed to be examined. Fortunately, Reece had not experienced any TM joint pain or clicking—yet.

As I explained what Reece was dealing with, he and his mom started to understand the relationship between a healthy mouth and other areas of the body. They began to see that a healthy mouth had direct correlation with airway breathing and TM joints. While they were happy to hear that we were getting to the source of Reece's problems, they were a little overwhelmed with all of the relationships—and with the course of therapy that would be involved in fixing his issues.

Feeling overwhelmed is a common experience when I inform patients that they have problems associated with obstructed breathing. That's because few dentists and physicians connect these dots, so patients haven't heard of these issues being associated with each other. It's also a lot of information and education to try to absorb all at once. But I always comfort patients by telling them not to worry: corrective therapy for sleep disorders and TM joints is a journey. It doesn't happen overnight, and we don't move forward until everyone involved understands the concepts and is comfortable with the journey to better breathing, optimal dentistry, and overall better health.

Just as Reece was, some patients are apprehensive about moving into oral appliance therapy. It can be costly and, for some patients, uncomfortable. If need be, a less costly, temporary appliance can be fabricated to give the patient a "trial run" of appliance fit and tolerance. That allows the patient to "test drive" the appliance and get a real feel for and appreciation of the benefits of appliance therapy.

# DAN—INSTANTLY FEELING AND SLEEPING BETTER

As soon as we delivered Dan's day and night appliances, he felt much better right away. When he came in for his two week follow up, my patient concierge greeted him and asked if he had been away for a spa retreat! He looked like a new man, the dark circles were gone, there was a spring in his step and a sparkle in his eye. He even told me that he had started to dream again, which is a sign that he was entering into the deeper, more restorative phase of sleep, rather than constantly waking before entering that phase. In fact, he was having fewer waking episodes, so much so that he was waking up in the morning feeling much more refreshed. His posture improved as well, and he was able to walk upright again.

As I write this book, we are about to begin weaning Dan off his daytime appliance. Once he is successful at that, we will then begin the cosmetic portion of his treatment to address the appearance of his front teeth.

---

Dan shares his experience about treatment at:
**https://vimeo.com/270695810**

---

Now let's take a deeper dive into what it means to ensure the mouth is healthy and has a strong foundation on which to provide cosmetic treatment.

# *Quick Quiz*

1.  What is MNRT and how does it help get to the root cause of a dental problem?

2.  What is the difference between restorative and cosmetic dentistry?

3.  Name three questions asked during a smile analysis questionnaire.

4.  Name five problems that may be addressed by a smile makeover.

5.  Name two benefits of an allograft.

# CHAPTER SIX

# GETTING YOUR ORAL FUNCTION BACK

Now let's get back to Reece who came into my office with badly broken-down back teeth. Now, as you may recall, he was young, a twenty-one-year-old, soon-to-be a college graduate.

His teeth were likely broken down for several reasons.

First, I believe there was a genetic component. I had restored his mom's teeth more than eight years prior with beautiful porcelain crown work to cover teeth that were soft. Why do I refer to her teeth as "soft"? Because they were very susceptible to tooth breakage, the cause of which can be a real challenge to determine. Again, with Reece, the problem could be genetics, or he could have an imbalance in the pH in his saliva. Or the problem might be a combination of both genetics and pH imbalance. As I mentioned in chapter 4, low pH diminishes the body's ability to heal.

What I suspect is that Reece has a version of a dental condition known as *amelogenesis imperfecta* (AI), although that has never been formally diagnosed. AI is a disorder of tooth development. This condition causes teeth to be discolored, pitted or grooved, and prone to rapid wear and breakage. He also clenches and grinds his teeth when he sleeps, which indicates that he can't breathe through his nose at night.

## RESTORE TEETH FIRST

The primary reasons I see patients for restorative work include cracks, decay, infection, or excessive wear.

I can speak from a patient point of view about the first of these reasons because I have suffered from having two cracked teeth in my mouth.

The first one occurred when I was in my early fifties. I cracked a tooth and it was sensitive to cold for months. But I ignored the sensitivity because I didn't think it hurt enough to do something about it. *Maybe it's just temporary pain*, I thought. *Maybe it will go away.* I was trying to rationalize my dental situation the way most of my patients rationalize their dental situations away. Kudos to those patients who come into my office as soon as cold sensitivity starts to bother them.

My avoidance behavior led me down a very painful road. One night, I decided to have a glass of red wine. As soon as the wine touched my tooth, I saw stars! The pain was unbelievable and unbearable. My whole body started to sweat. The four Advil I then ingested couldn't work fast enough. I recorked the bottle of wine and called it a night. Eventually, most of the pain subsided, and the next morning, I called Joe Chikvashvili. Joe is not only a good friend but also a truly excellent endodontist (root canal specialist). I reached out to him to see if could find room in his early-morning schedule to treat my cracked tooth.

Joe took an x-ray of the tooth and, based on it and other tests, he thought the tooth could be saved. The root canal was performed, and I felt much better—for the time being. The next day I had a dental colleague fabricate a provisional/temporary crown to protect the tooth. About a week or so after the crown was made for my tooth, I started to feel a dull discomfort upon chewing. Again, I tried to rationalize the pain. I thought maybe it was just part of the healing process of the root canal, so I gave it more time to heal.

As weeks progressed, the dull ache did not go away. I went back to Joe for an evaluation of the pain. He said that the tooth had probably been so badly cracked originally that the crack was causing an abscess below the gums and underlying bone. The tooth had to be extracted.

After the area healed, following the extraction, an implant was placed. A crown was then placed over the implant; a tiny screw connected the crown to the implant.

The other tooth fractured a few months before I began writing this book. With this one, I did not feel the tooth crack. I just began noticing some pain while chewing food. It was the same dull, aching sensation that I had felt with the other tooth a few years prior. Again, I called my root canal friend, Joe, and this time, we decided to extract the tooth right away rather than go through a root canal procedure. After the area healed, I had a second dental implant. I'll talk about implants later in this chapter.

For now, let's look at some of the other types of restorative work that can be done to create a healthier mouth. These are often done before cosmetic work. Again, restorative dentistry is how dentists repair problems in the mouth, such as decay, fractures, deterioration, or problem restorative work previously done.

Examples of restorations include fillings, crowns, bridges, implants, and dentures. Let me explain each of these more in-depth.

**Fillings**. Most of the decay in teeth that I see comes from cavities in between the teeth. I like to call these areas of decay "flossing cavities," because they occur in between teeth where only floss can go. Flossing is more challenging than brushing because it's more difficult and takes more time to do correctly. Many of my patients tell me that they understand the importance of flossing, but they don't do it, because they just don't want to. To them I say, "That's okay. Without flossing, we'll be 'friends' in my dental office for a real long time."

Often a filling is the solution for a cavity. Fillings really do not protect teeth. They don't protect or repair cracks either. All they do is fill spaces that were once filled with decay.

Fillings are the most common type of dental restoration. Teeth can be filled with silver, gold, or tooth-colored plastic material called composite resin.

Amalgam (mercury fillings) are the "silver" fillings used more often in the past. Amalgam fillings are attached to teeth via undercuts in the tooth structure. They are, basically, wedged into the teeth. I'm not a big fan of amalgam fillings. I don't really place them these days, largely because doing so is more invasive to the tooth and because much better technology is now available.

That technology is tooth-colored filling material known as composite resin. Composite resin filling technology was first introduced to dentistry in the 1950s. The early challenges of those plastic resin materials were their strength properties, how long they would last, and color properties, or how well they matched the rest of the tooth. But tooth-colored fillings really emerged in the 1980s. That's when composite resin filling materials were designed to adhere to tooth structure chemically, not just mechanically (like amalgam). That chemical bonding meant that fillings no longer needed to be held in place by undercuts in the tooth structure. Chemical bonding is a much less invasive way to fill teeth and it is much more esthetic.

As tooth-colored fillings came into the new millennium, the

chemical bond strengthened. The filling material itself has also been made stronger and more esthetic looking. In most instances these days, it's pretty much impossible to differentiate between the filling and the rest of the tooth.

Composite resin restorative materials continue to evolve. Their physical properties are still improving as are their handling, polish, and color characteristics. Since their results today are consistently high-quality, I use composite resin throughout the mouth. The strength of the material I use depends on the location of the tooth in the mouth. The composite I use in the back teeth is stronger and more durable for biting and chewing than the composite resin I use in the front teeth. However, the stronger material doesn't polish up nearly as well. More esthetic composite is used on the front teeth because it polishes up well, but it doesn't have the overall strength. So, there's some give and take.

**Crowns**. Crowns are tooth-shaped caps that are placed over teeth to restore them to their shape and size. Crowns are also used to hold bridges in place and to cover implants.

Crowns are really the only way to protect teeth from the forces that can cause them to crack and wear down over time. Crowns don't repair cracks, but they protect them from getting worse. When patients come into my office for their hygiene recare (or continuing care) appointment, I look for cracks in all their teeth. If I find one that could lead to further destruction (which cracks commonly do), I suggest a cap or crown on the tooth to protect it. That can reduce the chance that the patient will need root canal therapy and/or an extraction later on. I can't tell you how many times a patient has said to me, "Okay, Doc, so I have cracked teeth. But they don't hurt me. Can't we just watch them for a while?" To that, I reply, "Watch them? Watch them get worse? Not in my mind. I've walked that walk twice to no avail. Let's protect these cracked teeth by encapsulating them with crowns."

While many older ceramic crowns are stronger than natural tooth structure and/or enamel, technology in dental ceramics is developing at a rapid pace, constantly producing new materials for the restoration of a single tooth.

Until the 1980s, the crown of choice was made out of porcelain material that was baked onto a metal substructure. That metal core shows up over time and creates a disconcerting, very visible dark line at the gum line. Still, it was the most esthetic and strongest type of full coverage crown in its day.

In the 1990s and onward, the challenge was to make very strong, yet esthetically pleasing, all-porcelain/ceramic crowns that did not need any of the metal substructure. All-ceramic surrounding crowns—or crowns that cover the entire exposed surface of the tooth—have become more common because they allow for esthetic possibilities that are too difficult to achieve with metal surrounding systems.

The ideal crown materials should be strong, fit exceptionally well, and have lifelike esthetic qualities. Today, we have those ceramics. They are strong, fit exceptionally well, and are extremely beautiful. There is no metal in these new ceramic materials and some are so strong that all-ceramic bridges are becoming routine. Currently, on second molars and wisdom teeth—the teeth toward the back of the mouth—I use zirconia most of the time because it's the strongest ceramic material. On first molars and premolars—teeth on the sides of the mouth—I use IPS e.max, a kind of ceramic that is not as strong as zirconia but is strong enough for those teeth and is more esthetic. On the front teeth, I'm currently using feldspathic porcelain, which is incredibly esthetic and strong enough to withstand the biting forces of the front teeth.

At the same time the ceramic dentistry has taken off, digital dentistry has been following suit. Before 2000, dentists took crown impressions with a goopy material that was placed in a tray that fit in the patient's mouth. The material molded to the patient's teeth and, once it stabilized, it was removed from the mouth and replicated the tooth. The mold created by the goop was poured in stone and, from these impressions, a lab technician fabricated an all-surrounding crown. This technique for crown impression is still being used by most practitioners today.

In my practice, instead of the goopy impression material, we can now scan teeth with a small camera, a technique known as intraoral scanning. The images from the camera are uploaded into a computer where the scanned tooth is used to design the crown. Once designed, this information gets transferred to a milling machine that cuts a crown out of a block of porcelain. The technology allows the patients to receive their crown the same day.

Some of the benefits of digital scanning are:

* **Time savings**. It takes significantly less time to take a digital impression than a conventional, goopy impression, freeing up valuable chair time. That's a plus for the patient and the dentist. The time savings are multiplied for dentists who combine intraoral scanning with in-office milling, as opposed to sending the scan to an outside dental lab. As I mentioned, having in-house milling capabilities allows patients to have their crown fabricated while they wait in the office.[67]

---

67  Sebastian Patzelt et al., "The Time Efficiency of Intraoral Scanners: An In-Vitro Comparative Study," *The Journal of the American Dental Association* 145, no. 6 (June 2014): 542-551.

- **Convenience**. Intraoral scanning eliminates the mess of traditional, goopy impression materials, which many patients dislike.

- **Accuracy**. Studies have shown that intraoral scanning captures the surfaces of teeth more accurately than conventional impressions, leading to a better fitting restoration. Since fewer adjustments are needed, the appointment to place the crown is also shorter, which helps improve the patient's experience.[68]

**Bridges.** These restorations are designed to bridge the gap created by one or more missing teeth. Bridges can be anchored on either side by crowns and cemented into place. With a bridge, the teeth on either side of the missing tooth must first be prepared by taking away at least one millimeter to one and a half millimeters of structure around each tooth. Then we fabricate a bridge restoration that is made of crowns for each of those adjacent teeth, bridged by a "tooth" in the middle to fill the gap.

There are also temporary, removable bridges, known as nesbits, that clasp onto adjacent teeth. I'm not a fan of these because they're not stable. They don't give the existing teeth any occlusal support. They can also collect a lot of food and plaque around them, which leads to gum recession, over time, and they can even loosen the adjacent teeth that they clasp onto.

**Dentures.** Also, a restorative option for missing teeth, dentures are a removable replacement for missing teeth and surrounding tissues. They are made of acrylic resin, sometimes combined with metal attach-

---

68   Guillermo Pradies et al., "Clinical Evaluation Comparing the Fit of All-Ceramic Crowns Obtained from Silicone and Digital Intraoral Impressions," *Journal of Dentistry* 43, no. 2 (February 2015): 201–208.

ments. Complete or full dentures replace all the teeth. While they are often made as a removable option, they can also be fixed or secured to dental implants for better stability. Partial dentures are considered when some natural teeth remain. Partials are retained either by metal clasps attached to natural teeth or by implants with partial denture implant attachments. Those retained with clasps are removable. Those retained with implants are fixed.

People who have no teeth—lack of teeth is known as edentulism—are skeptical of dental treatments because of previous bad experiences. The most frequently reported overall denture complaint among this group is pain in the mandibular arch (lower jaw).[69] These patients frequently have high expectations regarding the ability to chew food with their new dentures. Unfortunately, the maximum biting force possible with both upper and lower dentures does not exceed one-fifth of the amount generated by natural teeth.[70]

**Implants**. Serving as replacement tooth roots, implants are small screws made of titanium or zirconia that are placed into the site of the missing tooth. The implant is then covered with a replacement called a crown.

Today, more than five million implants are placed every year and that number is growing, fueled in part by the needs of aging patients from generation X and the baby boomer generation.[71] In fact, the number of people with missing teeth will increase to more than 200

69   Veijo Lassila. Irma Holmlund, and Kalervo K. Koivumaa, "Bite Force and Its Correlations in Different Denture Types," *Acta Odontologica Scandinavica* 43, no. 3 (July 1985): 127–132.

70   Charles Gibbs et al., "Limits of Human Bite Strength," *The Journal of Prosthetic Dentistry* 56, no. 2 (August 1986): 226–229.

71   "Dental Implants Facts and Figures," American Academy of Implant Dentistry, accessed October 31, 2018, https://www.aaid.com/about/Press_Room/Dental_Implants_FAQ.html.

million during the next fifteen years.[72]

Not surprisingly, more dentists are acquiring education and training on how to place implants, believing that to be the new standard of care when compared with a traditional solution such as a bridge or dentures. As a patient, you need a dentist who will take the time to share with you details about the advantages of implant therapy if that is presented as an option for missing teeth.

To increase biting force and denture stability, full dentures can be secured by dental implants. This type of restoration is being advertised as "all-on-four," meaning all of the teeth in the arch of the denture are screwed into four implants. They are also advertised as "teeth-in-a-day." Both ideas are pushing the dental restorative envelope, in my opinion. What if one or two implants fail for one reason or another? If they fail, the whole case fails.

When placing implants as dentures, I usually place at least five implants in the upper jaw, and four in the lower jaw, although I prefer to place six in the upper jaw and five in the lower jaw. The more implants to support the long-span prostheses, the better. Having more implants is the best dental insurance available for patients missing numerous teeth, or all their teeth.

The edentulism patient needs more implants in the upper jaw than the lower jaw because the upper jaw bone is less dense. Whether patients are missing a few teeth or just one tooth, the replacement solution is either a bridge to span the space, which involves adjacent teeth, or a dental implant in the space, leaving the adjacent teeth alone. The latter of these gets my vote every time.

When a patient prefers a bridge over an implant, cost is usually the issue. Sometimes, however, the decision is based on a phobia, or if

---

72  "Facts & Figures," American College of Prosthodontists, accessed October 31, 2018, https://www.gotoapro.org/facts-figures/.

surgery poses a health risk. In these cases, bridgework is the restorative treatment plan of choice.

Again, restorative work is done before cosmetic work; I do esthetics last. If the patients have decay, periodontal disease, or missing teeth, I treat those issues first. The thought of putting veneers on upper front teeth when the patients have rampant decay and broken teeth in the back of their mouths makes me cringe.

At times, I work with other providers such as periodontists or oral surgeons to perform some of the complex components of implantology. However, as I mentioned in chapter 5, I also do bone and gum grafting, so most of the needs associated with an implant I address in-house.

## REECE'S OUTCOME

Remember Reece at the beginning of the chapter? He represents why good oral health is so important before beginning cosmetic treatment. In fact, one of Reece's premolars was so broken down that it was unable to be restored. That tooth had to be extracted and, after it heals, a dental implant will be placed in the space. I will place beautiful, ceramic crowns on most of Reece's teeth to protect them from further destruction. I'm waiting for him to make an appointment with an ENT to explore his sleep disordered breathing issue.

# *Quick Quiz*

1. Name three types of restorative treatment.

2. Name one of the materials used for crowns today.

3. What are three benefits of digital scanning?

4. What are dental implants?

# CHAPTER SEVEN

# ACHIEVING THE ULTIMATE OUTCOME

The word *ultimate* is defined as "the best achievable or imaginable of its kind." In esthetic dentistry, this definition can be extended to "the best achievable or manageable of its kind—for the patient." That means that what I, the dentist, perceive to be the ultimate esthetic outcome for patients might not align with the ultimate esthetic outcome of their victory—in other words, what they view as their ultimate smile.

A case in point is that of Margaux, who was twenty-six years old when she first sought treatment from me for esthetic dentistry on her four upper front teeth. She told me she wanted to improve her smile.

She had chairside bonding done on her front teeth some years prior but had never liked the way the treatment turned out.

To determine exactly what we needed to do to achieve Margaux's victory, we started with a smile analysis questionnaire that included ten questions. Here are the questions and Margaux's answers.

**Question:** Do you feel uncomfortable or self-conscious about your smile?

**Answer:** Yes.

**Question:** Do you cover your mouth when you talk or smile?

**Answer:** No.

**Question:** Are your teeth in straight alignment?

**Answer:** Yes.

**Question:** Do you wish your teeth were whiter?

**Answer:** Yes.

**Question:** Do you like the shape of your teeth?

**Answer:** No.

**Question:** Are your teeth chipped?

**Answer:** Yes.

**Question:** Can you see dark restorations in your teeth that bother you?

**Answer:** Yes.

**Question:** Do you have old crowns, bridges, and fillings that you don't like seeing?

**Answer:** Yes.

**Question:** Are you interested in human Botox or liquid facelift?

**Answer:** Yes.

**Question:** What would you like your smile to look like?

**Answer:** Margaux left this last answer blank, but during the initial consultation we were able to come to an understanding as to what she wanted her smile to look like.

At her initial consultation, we performed all the necessary x-rays to make a proper diagnosis.

We also took photographs of her teeth, and she and I looked at her photographs together as she pointed out all of her concerns. Among them was the fact that her bonded teeth were a different color than her natural teeth, her two front teeth didn't match (one was longer than the other and the shorter one was wider than the longer one), she didn't care for the shape of her bonded teeth, and there was a space known as a black triangle at the gum line between her two upper front teeth.

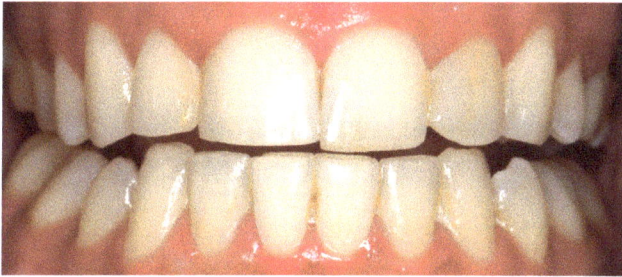

To my mind, the treatment plan for Margaux was extremely straightforward. Her ultimate smile could be achieved with four gorgeous porcelain veneers. I planned to strip the old bonding off her teeth and make an impression for four veneers. I also suggested that she consider letting me perform a gingivectomy to raise the gum tissue around all four teeth and expose more tooth structure in order to reduce the "gumminess" of her smile.

But as soon as I mentioned porcelain veneers to Margaux, she said, "No thank you."

For her, the ultimate outcome was to remove the old chairside bonding and replace it with the same treatment. Only, this time, she wanted it to look amazing. She also agreed to the gingivectomy procedure.

To ensure she understood the difference between bonding and porcelain veneers, I explained both to her. Bonding is a microscopically porous plastic, so it stains slowly over time depending on how much coffee, tea, dark soda, and red wine has been ingested. Porcelain veneers are like glass. Any stain that the porcelain veneers pick up gets brushed and polished away. The porcelain veneer deal breaker for Margaux was that some tooth structure—albeit it was ever so slight—would have to be removed to make the porcelain products fit and look natural. The chairside bonding would not require tooth structure to be removed.

While she understood that veneers might look better, she wanted the least invasive procedure. So new esthetic chairside bonding was Margaux's ultimate esthetic outcome.

The next step was to take two sets of study models. As I mentioned in chapter 5, these are casts of the patient's teeth. One set of casts represented her "before" teeth, and the other set was for the fabrication of the diagnostic wax-up to create her new teeth.

Some of the concerns I had in Margaux's case included making her four front teeth symmetrical. I also wanted to ensure they did not appear too wide. And I wanted them to look nice once the gum tissue was raised. In addition, I wasn't sure whether doing only the four front teeth would be enough. Would we also have to consider adding bonding material to Margaux's canine and eye teeth?

All these questions were worked out with the wax-ups (see photos). Upon completion of the wax-ups, I determined that I did not need to add composite bonding to the canines, since they did not need correcting. The gingivectomy for raising the gum tissue around all four teeth made the teeth look more esthetically harmonious in Margaux's smile. The teeth lengths and shapes were also more harmonious with her new smile than with her previous look. I showed her the wax-up along with her "before" model, so she could see what was in store for her. She was thrilled.

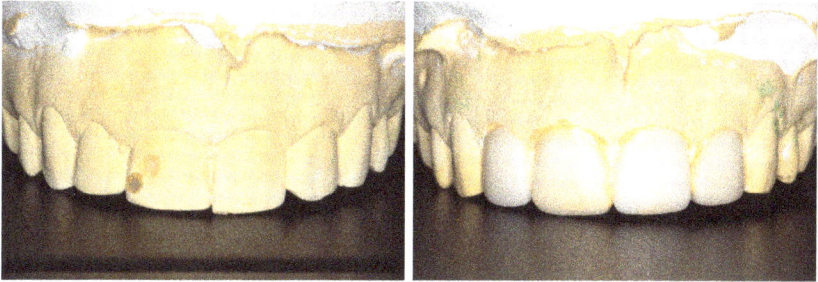

BEFORE                    AFTER

In preparation for her esthetic makeover, I fabricated an incisal jig of the wax-up. This jig is made from a putty that starts off soft and moldable. I place it over the edges of all the teeth that are being treated, along with a few of the teeth farther back on each side of the mouth, for stability.

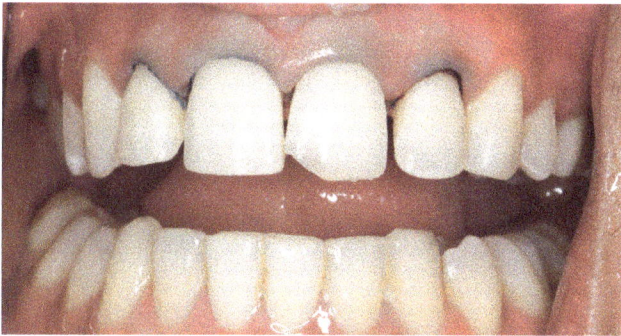

OLD BONDING REMOVED

After the old bonding is stripped away from the teeth, I place composite bonding in the incisal guide, which is then placed on the patient's teeth, positioning the bonding on and around the teeth in the ideal position. The bonding is then hardened using an LED light.

Once I have the edging of the new bonding on the existing teeth, I can add more bonding farther "up" the teeth toward the gum line.

After I place all the composite bonding, I do the gingivectomy. I finish off by polishing all of the bonding, making sure that all of the teeth are smooth, flossable, and gorgeous.

## COSMETIC DENTISTRY OPTIONS

As was the case with Margaux, many patients come to me because they are unhappy with another practitioner's work. That seems to be the most common reason patients seek me out.

For instance, another patient, Jennifer, came to me with the chief complaint that her bonded front tooth kept coming off. For her, victory would be a nice-looking bonded front tooth that would stay put. She told me that her previous dentist had repaired her chipped front tooth with bonded composite resin and that it had chipped off seven times in two months. Talk about patient frustration! After a thorough examination of her dental situation, I looked her in the eyes and said, "I can help you. I promise this new esthetic bonded restoration will stay repaired for a very long time." What's "long" in the dental-bonding world? About seven to ten years, not seven to ten days.

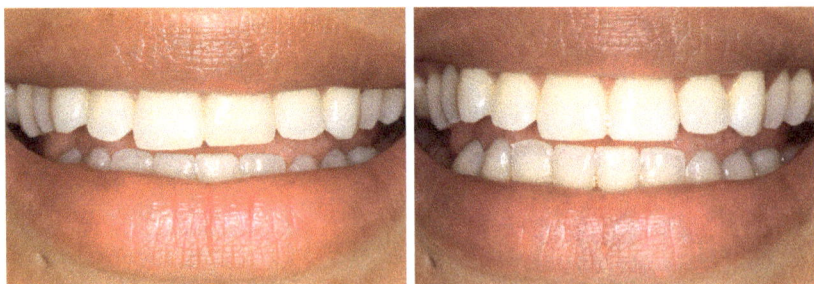

BEFORE                    AFTER

Another reason people seek cosmetic dentistry is to close unsightly spaces between teeth and repair broken, chipped, and discolored teeth in the smile zone. The smile zone includes all the patient's teeth that can be seen during a big smile, as when someone smiles at a really funny joke.

People also seek cosmetic dentistry to address the color of their teeth. They often try to whiten, using the rinses, gels, and strips that they find in pharmacies and markets, but they end up dissatisfied with the results. They want whiter teeth than they can get with those over-the-counter products. And they want their teeth to stay white longer. Their next option is in-office whitening, which I'll explain in greater detail later in this chapter. Sometimes the stain on the teeth is so deep—what dentists call intrinsic, that even in-office whitening won't do the trick. That's when it's time to discuss porcelain veneers or bonded composite veneers.

Let's look at some of these cosmetic dentistry options in detail.

**Bonded composite resin veneers**. As I mentioned previously, bonded composite resin veneer, in simple terms, is a plastic. It's a soft malleable material in its packaged form. Once the practitioner prepares the tooth (or teeth) in question, the material is placed in the mouth and sculpted into the shape of a tooth (or teeth). An LED light is then shined on the newly sculpted material, which starts a chemical reaction in the resin that makes it harden and bond to the existing tooth structure.

Advantages to composite resin veneers include:

- **Abrasion or wear considerations**. Many composite resins wear much like natural tooth structure and do not cause wear of opposing teeth.

- **Darkly stained teeth**. Composite resin can cover dark coloring on teeth while retaining their vital appearance.

- **Conservation of tooth structure**. Tooth preparation for composite resin veneers can be more conservative than for porcelain alternatives because composite resin does not require 0.5 millimeters of thickness as porcelain does. Composite resin can be much thinner in spots and still function well and look good.

- **Fabrication**. Composite resin veneers can be fabricated in the office, chairside, and often the treatment can be done in one visit.

**Chairside repairs**. These can be made easily, with the same bonded, light-cured material as used for composite resin veneers.

**Veneers**. Previously, I discussed the difference between bonded veneers and porcelain veneers. Let's dig a little deeper into porcelain veneers.

The porcelain laminate veneer was introduced in 1983.[73] There are different types of dental porcelain. The most esthetic porcelain is called "feldspathic" porcelain. When made properly, this porcelain is strong and has an excellent fit, and lifelike esthetic qualities. This is the porcelain veneer of choice for most esthetic dentists. Other porcelain veneer compositions might be a little stronger but not nearly so esthetic.

To prepare a tooth for a porcelain veneer, tooth reduction is necessary. The tooth structure needs to be reduced at least one millimeter all the way around to guarantee adequate porcelain strength against all chewing movement and forces. The prepared shape of each tooth needs to be smooth, rounded, and flowing. Sharp corners must be avoided because they create fracture lines in the porcelain over time.

Porcelain veneers are bonded in place with a resin cement, which, along with other adhesive dental materials, creates a very strong, long-lasting bond to tooth structure. I inform my patients that a properly

---

73    Núbia Pavesi Pini et al., "Advances in Dental Veneers: Materials, Applications, and Techniques," *Clinical, Cosmetic and Investigational Dentistry* 4 (2012): 9-16, https://www. ncbi.nlm.nih.gov/pmc/articles/PMC3652364.

placed porcelain veneer can last up to fourteen years.

Usually, before we do a big veneer case, we strongly suggest whitening the natural teeth that are not being veneered. Once the natural teeth are whitened, we match the new veneers to the newly whitened natural teeth.

**Whitening**. Most esthetic dentists offer two kinds of teeth-whitening treatment: in-office and take-home. The in-office treatment takes about an hour and a half in the dental chair and consists of four, fifteen-minute bleach applications. To protect the gums during this procedure, the gum tissue is covered with a resin so that only the teeth are exposed to the whitening bleach. The take-home system consists of upper and lower dental-arch whitening trays that are customized to fit the patient's teeth. We take upper and lower arch molds to fabricate these whitening trays. A very small amount of whitening gel is placed in each tray; it doesn't take a lot of whitening gel to get great results. I suggest to my patients that they wear these trays for about thirty minutes daily for two weeks. I have found that the combination of in-office and take-home whitening techniques achieve the finest whitening results.

**Botox and dermal fillers**. *The Oxford Dictionary* describes Botox as a "drug prepared from the bacterial toxin botulin, used medically to treat certain muscular conditions and cosmetically remove wrinkles by temporarily paralyzing facial muscles."

In my practice, I give Botox injections to remove or soften forehead wrinkles, the lines created above the nose and between the eyes in the glabellar area of the face. When I ask a patient to look stern, those muscles can create the deep lines that look like the number eleven. That's why we refer to these wrinkles as "eleven lines."

Botox can also soften crow's feet lines, which are at the outer edges of the eyes, and it can help remove lines around the mouth. Although the mouth lines are sometimes called "smoker's lines," even nonsmokers can get them by sucking on straws and water bottles, over time. All the muscles that cause these wrinkles or lines can be corrected and/or softened by Botox.

Dermal fillers help to diminish lines and restore volume and fullness in the face. As we age, our faces naturally lose subcutaneous fat (fat under the skin). That causes the facial muscles to work closer to the skin's surface, so smile lines and crow's feet become more apparent. The facial skin also stretches a bit, adding to the loss of facial volume. In addition to aging, other factors that affect the facial skin include sun exposure, heredity, and lifestyle.

I use dermal fillers in my office to plump lips, enhance shallow contours of the face, and soften facial creases and wrinkles. Sometimes I use a combination of Botox and dermal fillers to correct deep lines in the face.

The type of filler used depends on where the treatment is on the face because different fillers are made of different-sized particles. For instance, in the lips, which tend to get thinner with age, I use a filler with a very small particle size to avoid lumpiness.

A fabulous dermal filler procedure that I call a "liquid facelift" contains larger-sized particles. It is used to plump up the cheeks. When the cheeks are lifted, the skin folds by the nose also soften. A liquid facelift is a nice procedure that creates a beautiful correction to a large area of the face.

Remember that Botox and dermal fillers are short-term treatments for facial aging. Repeat applications of Botox are typically needed every six to eight months. Dermal fillers need to be repeated every year or so, for long-term benefits.

**Invisalign**. In my practice, we treat quite a few patients with Invisalign, the clear plastic aligners or trays that slowly straighten teeth, much as braces do. Both braces and Invisalign were designed to straighten teeth while improving the patient's smile and overall oral health. Invisalign allows me to treat many cases, some of which are straightforward and include crowded teeth, dental arch expansions, and teeth straightening.

However, I'm not an orthodontist, so I don't offer treatment with traditional braces, and with Invisalign, I don't do complex cases that involve a lot of movement or corrections to align the teeth. When patients have very complex orthodontic issues, I refer them to an orthodontist. For instance, molars that don't line up properly against each other when the teeth are closed present a complex issue that an orthodontist needs to address. I also refer patients to an orthodontist if, for instance, they have an underbite: their lower front teeth are out farther than their upper front teeth when they close their mouth. I also refer them if they have an open bite: their back teeth touch during a bite, but they have a gap between their upper and lower front teeth.

Invisalign first came into favor around the year 2000, so this treatment does not have the same history as braces, but I've seen some incredible results using the Invisalign system of aligners. Invisalign is designed to be—you guessed it—invisible. The aligner trays are made of smooth, comfortable, and clear plastic that is worn over the teeth to subtly and very gently move them into place. We use x-rays to take photographs and impressions of the patient's mouth, which are sent to Invisalign. The company's lab technicians use the materials to create a precise 3-D image of the patient's teeth that is used as the model for configuring the sequence of the aligner trays.

The aligners must be worn for at least twenty-two hours per day. The patients are given a series of aligners to take home, and they switch out to the next aligner in the series every ten days. Treatment usually lasts, on average, from six to eighteen months, depending on the patients' needed outcome.

Regardless of the tool used to straighten teeth (braces or Invisalign), the patients must understand before treatment begins that they need to wear a retainer at night for the rest of their life in order to keep their teeth straight. If the patients do not comply with this etched-in-stone rule, their teeth will relapse, returning to the crooked state they were in before treatment.

**Laser contouring**. In previous chapters, I mentioned performing gum contouring to even out gum tissue and create a more symmetric smile. I perform gum contouring using a laser when patients have excess gum tissue that extends down their teeth and makes them appear disproportionately small. I also use it at the end of treatment when patients have an uneven gum line, because that can cause teeth to look uneven, irregularly shaped, or crooked.

Gum contouring is a quick and relatively painless cosmetic procedure that requires only a local anesthetic. While there is some discomfort following the procedure, the results once the gums are healed are always an improvement.

## DIGITAL DENTISTRY

Over the past thirty years that I've been practicing, the dental profession has experienced an exciting amount of technological growth. Digital dentistry has been broadly defined as "any dental technology or device that incorporates digital or computer-controlled components in contrast to that of mechanical or electrical alone."[74]

---

74 Paul L. Childe, Jr., "Digital Dentistry: Is This the Future of Dentistry?" *Dental Economics*, October 1, 2011, https://www.dentaleconomics.com/articles/print/volume-101/issue-10/features/digital-dentistry-is-this-the-future-of-dentistry.html.

A digital office is a modern, computerized office. For technology in digital dentistry to be considered a clear advantage and introduced into a practice, it must offer three benefits: deliver an enhanced patient experience; contribute more predictable, high-quality treatment outcomes; and improve practice efficiency and productivity. If a technology offers all three of these benefits, then it certainly behooves dental practitioners to consider adding it to their practices.

One of the areas of dentistry in which dramatic changes have occurred is digital radiography—dental x-rays, intraoral cameras, and external oral cameras are all digital today. I've used digital radiography in my office for at least the past twenty years. It was an easy decision to bring digital radiography into my office. Why? Less x-ray radiation to the patient. That was first and foremost a factor in my decision to switch to digital. Digital x-rays deliver practically no radiation to the patient; the patient is exposed to more radiation walking outside for any length of time on a sunny day.

Another minor advantage of digital x-rays is the development process. With digital, there's no x-raying film and dipping it into chemicals of developer and fixer. That was a messy, smelly process that took up to twenty minutes to develop a full-mouth series of x-rays. With digital x-rays, we take a picture and it pops up on the computer screen in seconds. Believe it or not, I know many dental colleagues who still use the antiquated film-and-developer x-ray system.

In addition to minimal radiation and faster processing of the images—which means significantly less time in the chair for the patient—digital radiography creates better images to use in treatment planning. Since the images are digital, they are much easier to organize and store, helping to improve the efficiency of treatment for patients. Although going digital can be costly, the advantages of digital radiography far outweigh any limitations imposed by cost.

Within the scope of digital radiography in my practice, we also have cone beam computed tomography (CBCT). Conventional and digital x-rays produce two-dimensional representations, meaning only height and width are represented in the pictured object. CBCT, however, allows us to see what's going on all around the scanned object—in other words, in three dimensions: height, width, and depth. CBCT is an exciting technology that has been rapidly growing in usage because of several factors: the scanner costs less today than when it was originally introduced to the market, the number of general dentists placing implants has risen, it uses less radiation compared to conventional CT scans, and it has been rapidly adopted by universities and medical and dental specialists.

As I mentioned, I am among those dentists now placing implants, and I find the CBCT to be an invaluable tool because its effectiveness and accuracy is unparalleled. I also use the CBCT digital technology to determine whether a patient has a sleep disordered breathing problem or a TMD problem because the CBCT gives me a 3-D image of the airway and the jaws joints.

Digital photography is also part of a modern practice. Of course, digital is pretty much the worldwide standard in photography today. I'm always taking digital photographs of my patients' mouths with an intraoral camera, which is much smaller than a conventional camera, allowing it to fit inside the mouth and get close-up views of each tooth and even very small oral problems.

Finally, in the previous chapter, I explained how we scan teeth with a digital scanner, send the information to a computer, and then use that information to design crowns and bridges in-office. Or we send the information to a lab and have the lab technicians design and fabricate the crown or bridge. We also have the digital technology to scan dental implants. Scanning teeth and implants is becoming easier and faster and better for the patient. With digital dentistry now in the picture, it is not a question of whether digital scanning will replace conventional, goopy impression taking, but when.

## MARGAUX'S AMAZING OUTCOME

Now for Margaux's outcomes.

When I gave Margaux the mirror at the end of the three-and-a-half-hour appointment, she smiled with amazement and excitement. I was also very happy—and relieved—that I had exceeded her expectations.

In truth, porcelain veneer fabrication would have looked just as nice and with very little staining long-term. A porcelain-veneer appointment would have been less labor intensive for me, since bonding is a more intricate procedure than porcelain veneering. But what's most important is that we more than met Margaux's ultimate outcome. We changed her smile, all in one appointment.

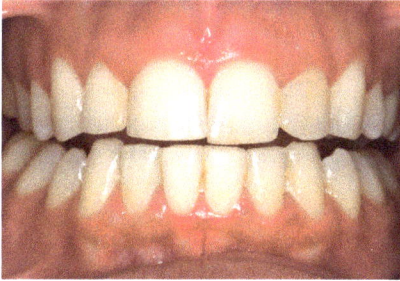 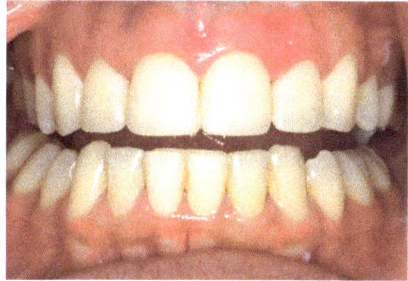

BEFORE                                              AFTER

# *Quick Quiz*

1.  What is the difference between bonding and veneers?

2.  Name three advantages of composite resin veneers.

3.  Name two areas of the face where Botox or dermal fillers can help.

4.  What are three benefits that digital dentistry must offer?

# CHAPTER EIGHT

# WHAT MOTIVATES YOU?

There are two big hurdles affecting most dentists and their practices outside their offices. These hurdles also affect patients' decisions on choosing the ideal dental practice that can meet their needs. Both hurdles revolve around money: dental insurance and corporate dentistry.

Dental insurance companies are in the business of signing up individuals and dental practices for their coverage and then sending these prospective patients only to those dentists who have signed up for their discounted plans.

In this system, to quote a good friend and mentor of mine, Scott Manning, "The patient can see no value because they're taught that dentistry has no value. In their system. Every dentist is considered to be like every other dentist. They're all the same."[75] These insurance companies do not pay more for the skills that I have versus a dentist down the street who has just started in practice or who has not been devoted to honing skills. Insurance doesn't take into account that I've undergone years of accredited, continuing

---

75 Scott J. Manning, *Mastering the Lost Art of Patient Retention: How to Turn Your Patient Base into a Never-Ending Gold Mine*, (Franklin, Tennessee: Dental Success Today), 2018.

education beyond my initial training.

Scott goes on to say, "If the patient is trained by the insurance industry, they're taught the concept of discounting, and that the treatment is not necessary. Insurance companies try to play the doctor." What are these insurance companies teaching patients? Go for routine cleanings and then have any cavities filled. In other words, insurance companies are conditioning John Q. Public to be very emergency minded. They teach people to wait until "it's broken" or "it hurts" before they seek treatment.

Day in and day out, my team at The Miller Center engages with the patients who want to know what is going on in their mouths. The team asks questions and educates them on why they need our service—and how it can be afforded. Along the way, the patient gathers insight as to why The Miller Center does not participate with any of the insurance companies.

Even the name *insurance company* is slightly misleading. It's not really insurance. It's more like a benefit. What other kind of insurance requires you to use it by the end of the calendar year or lose it? That use-it-or-lose-it "insurance" money, typically, adds up to about $1,500 to $2,000 per calendar year. How much is being taken out of your paycheck every month to pay for this "insurance"? It's costly, and more often than not, it's not worth the yearly benefit.

As I mentioned, the other hurdle is corporate dentistry. Their approach is, to quote my dear friend Scott again: "To take the patients in and spit them out. They do just enough to max out the insurance, and then they go on to the next patient. Basically, they are in cahoots with the insurance companies. They have ruined the reputation of care and service. Their approach downplays the integrity of dentistry. They do not have a relationship with patients, and often have a revolving door of dentists."

This is a fight that I am prepared to win every day. Our practice is about educating patients and establishing patient relationships. Our patients realize that our fees are based on our expertise, knowledge, customer service, and cutting-edge equipment. After all is said and done, it's really not about the money. People have to feel comfortable with the person treating them. If they are comfortable with us and the treatment we provide, they're going to stick to my dental practice like glue.

Again, it's all about relationships, and in my practice, that starts by asking patients, "What would be a victory for you?" That's how we begin to establish rapport with our patients. Then we take the time to educate patients about their treatment. We do this carefully, however, because we want patients to participate in their treatment planning so they will develop a sense of ownership. We've found that too much information can cause patients to stop listening. In fact, even at The Miller Center, occasionally, a patient won't come back after the initial consultation. Why? Well, there are several reasons why patients don't return to a dental practitioner after a first visit.

One reason is extenuating circumstances. For instance, in 2007, when the stock market crashed, people held onto their money. Some of them were forced to ask, "Should I get a crown for my broken tooth, or should I put bread on the table?" Some of the time, they opted to put bread on the table and go down the street where they could get a discounted crown for their broken tooth from Dr. X. Then, a few years later, they came back to me to redo the ill-fitting, irritating crown that Dr. X made.

Another reason is a lack of trust. As Scott states, "It's all about trust. Money moves to trust, to confidence, to certainty."

Patients also don't go back because they didn't feel the experience was personal. If you go someplace for a service and you don't feel that personal touch, you don't feel the person there to help you is listening or providing answers to your needs, do you want to go back?

A sense of authenticity is also important to patients. When they don't get that feeling through an interaction with a practice, it's usually because there is too much focus on the money and the insurance. Scott even advises that talking about money and insurance too soon when building a relationship can ruin any bond that may be established early on.

One last reason is that some dental practitioners don't make dentistry important enough for the patient to follow through. As Scott says, "If the patient doesn't feel like the treatment needs to be done now, they're not going to do it now." Dental practitioners sometimes give patients an excuse and teach them to delay treatment. I'm sure most of us have been in a dental chair during a dental examination and heard the phrase, "We'll put a watch on that tooth."

The real question is: What are we watching? Are we watching a small area of decay and waiting for it to get bigger and more extensive, eventually needing a bigger filling? Are we watching a little crack in a tooth and waiting for it to get so big that the tooth breaks so it then needs a root canal? Are we waiting until it needs to be restored with a post and core and a crown?

To all my dental colleagues, I send this request: I ask you to stop waiting and do more doing. To dental patients all over the world, I send this message: consider asking your dentist, *What are we watching?* Why not be more proactive and preventive and treat what the doctor has found in order to prevent the "watch" from getting worse?

The key to success in dentistry is, ultimately, doing what's right for the patients and keeping them engaged. Give them a reason to come back to the dental office. The more the patients come back, the more preventive care can be achieved to avoid any possible dental problems down the line of life. It's common sense: The mouth is part of the human body, and the human body gets older every day. Therefore, the mouth gets older every day. It follows that, as you age, more problems can begin to occur.

Scott asks the question, "What do people complain about when they go to the doctor? They talk about the fact that the doctor is spending no time with them, and the doctor knows nothing about them. There's nothing personal that happens at the visit. The number one complaint is that a doctor doesn't listen. The patient doesn't feel listened to."

How many times have I gone to the doctor's office, and the receptionist barely says hello, let alone makes eye contact with me? After I check in and the receptionist asks me, "What brings you in today?" I sit down and wait for twenty minutes to be brought into an examination room. Then, in the examination room, I sit for a good thirty minutes. The nurse, finally, enters the room and the first words out of the nurse's mouth are, "Hi, what brings you in today?" Obviously, there was little or no communication between the front office and the exam area in reference to my care. Again I give the nurse the reason for my visit, she takes my blood pressure, records my weight, and then tells me the doctor will be in soon. Another twenty minutes go while I sit in the exam room by myself with no engagement of any kind with anyone in the office.

Finally, the doctor comes in. What do you think are the first words out of the doctor's mouth? You guessed it: "What brings you in today?" I can't make this stuff up. Why would I, as a patient, ever want to come back to this office?

The doctor and staff must make the office visit personal. The team has to listen to each and every patient. In Scott's words, "The patients that a doctor wants … do not want the approach that insurance and corporations breed. Give them something different. Something personal."

That's what I want and need as a patient myself, and that's what we deliver at my practice: that personal touch. The conversations that I and my team have with patients are professional but friendly and authentic. But we want patients to be participants in their care. Patient engagement involves everything we do at The Miller Center for Dental Excellence and our Miller TMJ & Sleep Therapy Center.

Again, we begin by asking patients about their "victory," their main reason for visiting the office that day. Then, we go through the patients' medical history. The necessary x-rays and photographs are taken. We confirm the patients' goals and exceed their expectations. We share stories and testimonials.

As I mentioned earlier, we want to take care not to overwhelm patients with too much information. In other words, as Scott says, we don't want to "just dump all the treatment on (our patients) all at once." We don't want to hurry them into something so quickly that they don't know what's happening. As we go through the photographs, I often say something like such as, "Based on what we see, this is what I suggest that we do next." That's in answer to what may be the most common question I hear from patients: "What's next?" They rarely ask me, "How much treatment is left until we finish the total treatment plan?" They just want to know what's next. That's why we make complicated plans less overwhelming by cutting the treatment up into bite-sized pieces. In other words, how do you eat an elephant? The answer is: one piece at a time.

So, to recap: At The Miller Center, we know how important it is to find out each patient's goals and objectives and to share the objectives and recommendations for treatment. We know how important it is for every member of the team to be aware of each patient's "victory."

Why? So that our patients feel that the whole office is in tune with their visit and they will work with us to move forward with their priorities. It's when our patients feel that they are being treated almost as an extended part of our office family that we have true patient engagement. We know that treatment is not "all or nothing"; we can take each priority as it comes to help patients get back their smiles—and take back their lives.

# CONCLUSION

I started preparing for this book more than ten years before I wrote the words that you're reading now. In that initial effort, I wanted to write the perfect dental self-help book for everyone to read because I thought I had something to say. My intent at that time was to inform and educate. I started writing it with one of my patients, Margarethe Laurenzi, who I found had a talent and skill for writing. We put together what we both felt at the time was a nice, engaging manuscript.

Then life got in the way. In 2007, I divorced from two partners: my marriage of seventeen years came to an end, and my business partner of nine years "blew up" our dental practice.

Fast forward to 2017. My practice management coach, Scott Manning, explained to me the importance of writing a book. He said, "Craig, people want to hear what you have to say. You need to finish your book."

Scott gave me the contact information of a publishing company, Advantage Media Group, and I was introduced to my project editor, Regina Roths. Through Scott and the people at Advantage, I was able to flesh out and update my book. In the end, I was glad I took ten years off from the book project because I had more time to grow as a person and as a dental practitioner.

Dental technology has changed drastically over the past ten years, making today the perfect time to bring this book to fruition. Now, it's not just about writing the perfect self-help book to inform and educate about dentistry, it's also about offering information on improving patient outcomes—and improving lives, as a result.

With this book, I hope that I'm helping prospective patients decide on their dental outcomes. But I also hope that I'm helping dentists better understand how to achieve the best dental outcome for their patients. The secret? Working together. To achieve the best outcomes, dentists and patients must both think favorably about each and every dental experience.

I've talked about trust building, exchanging valued goals and expectations, and the importance of having constant, open dialog. By dialing in the dental experience leading up to the comprehensive clinical exam, dentists can give patients the answers they need to know in an empowering way so that they feel confident and comfortable enough to schedule and pay for their pathway to health.

As a patient, you should feel and absorb your dentist's philosophy even before you open your mouth. That starts by providing you with a good experience from the minute you enter the practice and should include concern for a healthy mouth, proper bite, proper breathing, strong dentition, a complete set of teeth, and a beautiful smile. Your dentist's philosophy should elevate your interest in dentistry and compel you to want more for yourself. And your dentist should tell you what the process is expected to be like and what your role in the whole experience will be. As a prospective patient, you should expect nothing less.

I hope you've found this book to be more than dental information and education. I hope that I've given you a better understanding of how the patient-doctor engagement can be empowering. I'm glad I figured this out with a little help from my friends along the way. If I have been able to give you one or two pearls in this book—if I have been able to help you enjoy your understanding of dentistry, or feel better about yourself—then writing it was worth the time. As the title of the book asserts, when you get back your smile, you get back your life—and I hope my book inspires you to do just that.

# ACKNOWLEDGMENTS

T hank you to my wife, Brenda. You are truly the love of my life and my biggest fan. You are not just a lovely wife—you are The Miller Center office manager, business manager, and the make-it-happen officer. I cherish our partnership and life together.

Thank you to my mother, Nora, for all of your love and support. With your PhD in linguistics, your literary prowess is second to none. You've raised a son who takes grammar very seriously.

Thank you to my father, Edwin, an ophthalmologist who was loved by all of his patients and placed the calling of health care professional in my DNA. You continue to inspire me to be the best doctor I can be.

Thank you to my sister, Leslie, and my brother, Andrew, brilliant physicians in their own right. Your dedication to your work keeps me wanting to learn more in health care. I couldn't have better siblings.

Thank you to my children and stepchildren, Janine, Dana, Kaitlyn, Cassie, and Dean. It has been wonderful and miraculous to watch all of you grow up to be such beautiful people. I love you! Look out world!

Thank you to Drs. Steven Olmos and Daniel Klauer. You've taken my dental learning and dental practice to another level of patient care.

You are leaders in your field of expertise, and learning from you has truly been an inspiration.

Thank you to Dr. Enoch Ng. A few years ago, you were one of my general practice residents and I was teaching you and your fellow residents at Newark Beth Israel Hospital. More years go by and now I'm learning from you! It's been exciting watching you develop into the amazing practitioner that you have become.

Thank you to my good friends and mentors, Scott Manning and Kevin Kowalke. You are a dynamic team that has been an incredible support system for me, personally, and for The Miller Center.

Lastly, thank you to my office team and patients at The Miller Center. I can't do what I do without you!

# ABOUT THE AUTHOR

Robert Craig Miller, raised in Short Hills, New Jersey—a suburb of Manhattan, New York—attended Lehigh University, where he started creating smiles as a cheerleader for the Lehigh Mountain Hawks football team.

After graduating from Lehigh, he earned his doctor of dental medicine degree (DMD) from The University of Medicine and Dentistry of New Jersey, now known as the Rutgers School of Dental Medicine. While attending dental school with five other students named Bob, he decided to go by his middle name, Craig.

After completing an advanced general dental practice residency at Mount Sinai Hospital in Manhattan, Dr. Miller became a fellow and master of the Academy of General Dentistry, having passed a comprehensive written exam and completed over 500 hours of continuing education courses in all dental disciplines. In addition, three years of intensive, hands-on oral implantology training led to his becoming a fellow of the International Congress of Oral Implantologists. Through extensive training at the Pankey Institute for Advanced Dental Education, Dr. Miller stays current with advances in dental technology and techniques in treating the entire system of facial joints, muscles, and teeth.

As a hybrid dentist who offers general, cosmetic, restorative, and surgical services, Dr. Miller remains intellectually curious about all aspects of improving the dental health of his patients. He is on staff at Saint Barnabas Hospital in Livingston, NJ, and at Newark Beth Israel Hospital in Newark, NJ, where he teaches dental residents restorative, implant, and advanced cosmetic dentistry, along with dental sleep medicine.

# CONTACT US

**The Miller Center for Dental Excellence
and The TMJ & Sleep Therapy Centre
of Metropolitan New Jersey**

22 Old Short Hills Road, Suite 206
Livingston, New Jersey, 07039
Phone: 973-533-0053
TheMillerCenter.com

www.ingramcontent.com/pod-product-compliance
Lightning Source LLC
Chambersburg PA
CBHW051436270326
41935CB00019B/1838